SIN, SEX, SCANDAL, AND DOCTORING

BILL LARKWORTHY

Front Cover: Adam and Eve. Lucas Cranach the Elder (1526).Courtesy Courtauld Institute, London

Back Cover: Bill Larkworthy and his wife, Maria, enjoying a glass of local wine on the terrace of their house in Provence. Photograph: Norbert Stiastny.

ISBN - 13: 978-1511920582
ISBN-10: 1511920580

DEDICATION

This book is dedicated to Maria, my wife and soulmate,
who looks after my every need, including patiently
handling my lamentable computing skills

CONTENTS

PREFACE

I THOUGHT THAT WHEN I WROTE MY MEMOIR... *DOCTOR LARK – the benefits of a medical education*... that's it, no more stories in me.' But, once bitten by the writing bug, the urge to put both index fingers to the keyboard lingered, grew, and like an itch, demanded scratching. So, I wrote this anthology about topics which interest me, and which I think, others will find diverting and amusing.

The ongoing male dominance on our planet taxes me and whilst ruminating about it I was spurred to review its origins and evolution. Obviously the male starts out with the advantage of being physically the stronger: he is the tough hunter-gatherer and she the weaker home-maker. Man, however, becomes even more dominant when the major religions come along; he assumed control because those religions, revealed to the divinely-inspired Christianity's first saints and prophets (all male), promoted male theocratic governance while elaborating male superiority in intellect and artistic skills.

I have included a few articles about some of my experiences as a young doctor, most of which can never be repeated, because the world in which I practised changed so much during the fifty years in which I wielded my stethoscope.

When I finished doctoring, over a decade ago, I retired to live in a fascinating corner of France, beautiful Provence, which is so full of history and lively stories that I felt bound to share a few.

Bill Larkworthy.

1. ALL SEX IS SINFUL

WHILE I WAS READING ACCOUNTS OF THE EARLY CHRISTIAN CHURCH'S teachings about sexual rights and wrongs I couldn't help thinking that had Christians followed those teachings to the letter they would have stopped reproducing, and Christianity would have extinguished itself.

As far as sex is concerned our saintly forebears were united in preaching that one sure path to eternal bliss is to avoid sex completely. Those wise and saintly teachers (all men, strangely enough) also taught that Woman is inferior to Man – a doctrine which was based on the Old Testament story of The Fall of Eve in The Garden of Eden.

At the beginning of the Middle Ages the Christian Church became established in a seriously troubled Rome and developed an all-powerful hierarchy. It took it upon itself to intrude into every aspect of the private lives of men and women and to punish those who did not conform to its rules. Aberrant sexual behaviour, as defined by the Bible and by the Elders of the Church, preoccupied Episcopal conferences in the early Middle Ages. The Church's control over what is a basic biological

1

function expanded after the 15th century when the Roman Catholic hierarchy declared that its bishops and priests must follow apostolic tradition by denying their natural instincts and have no physical contact with women, thus removing the possibility that the sacred elements of the Eucharist might be handled by hands which had recently handled the profane parts of a woman.

When, however, clerics were commanded to remain celibate and continent the Church's leaders ignored the fact that many early saints were married and indeed that the Prince of the Apostles, St Peter, was married and had a family when he became the first Pope. Cynics might say that the motive behind the Church's declaration was not spiritual, it was financial. When a married priest died his family inherited his worldly possessions, but if priests were not allowed to marry, Mother Church would be the benefactor.

The Age of Enlightenment, between the early 17th and the 19th centuries, saw loosening of the strict obedience to the Church's laws. In the next epoch, the Victorian era, the lay public itself, through its middle classes, re-implanted the notion that sexual activity, especially in men, was unclean – contrasting with today's approaches to sex and marriage which have swung so far from the rigid medieval and Victorian codes that there is now a bewildering state of 'anything goes'.

In the past Christians adapted their behaviour in accordance with the rules of the Church but times have changed and today the situation is reversed. Anglican clerics are finding difficulty in deciding how to adapt the Church to a world which is becoming more and more secular. In recent years Anglican priests unable to reconcile their beliefs with the ordination of women, or the acceptance of homosexuality and same-sex marriage, have converted to the Church of Rome. The Pope welcomed them and allowed married Anglican priests to remain married. In many countries the equality of sexes is defined in law but in spirit there is still some way to go. Within living memory homosexuality has been decriminalised in western countries, and in recent years many countries have legalised same-sex marriage; indeed sexual freedom of expression has reached such an over-the-top state that in 2013 a fashion mogul announced that he wished to marry his cat.

LIKE MOST OF MY GENERATION MY ATTITUDES TO LIFE AND SEX were implanted at an early age. I was born into an Anglican family; strictly low-church, no bells, no smells, and church attendance obligatory at least once every Sunday. To me it seemed that Sunday after Sunday our vicar thundered the same message from his pulpit: 'Eat, drink and be merry, for tomorrow you die!'

That was the favourite fear-inducing theme for the sermons of our vicar, the Reverend H G MacMaking. It surely hit the spot for little me, aged seven or eight, quaking as I gazed up at him. After waving his arms and working himself into a lather he would abruptly pause, gaze slowly, silently and deliberately around his petrified congregation... and then, grasping the edge of the pulpit, lean over and fix me, and only me, with a penetrating gaze and menacingly confide, 'This very day as you leave this House of God you could be hit by a bus and killed and then...,' in a voice rising and ringing with triumphalism, '... and then where would you be?' Indeed, where would I be? A question which has haunted me to this day.

That was in the parish church of my youth – St Jude, the patron saint of lost causes – in the ancient naval city of Plymouth. The Rev MacMaking instilled so much guilt in me that seven decades later if I catch myself having a laugh there is a twitch of unease in the back of my cranium. It took me many years to realise that Mr MacMaking was simply doing what the Christian Church has always commanded of its clerics... scare them, make them feel guilty and then offer salvation if they promise to behave.

ACCORDING TO JAMES USHER (1581-1656), BISHOP OF ARMAGH in Northern Ireland, the world began over six thousand years ago. He used the Bible for his calculations and came up with the year 4000BC, he added four years to take account of Herod's death; quite why escapes me. Bishop Usher was precise; he wrote that The Creation was completed at dusk on 23 October 4004BC.

Genesis, the First Book of the Old Testament of the Christian Bible, tells us that God's first human creation was a man, Adam. Then he took one of Adam's ribs and from it created a woman, Eve. He made them both in his own image and for a while all went well in the Garden of Eden. Went well that is, until the Devil in the form of the Serpent tempted Eve to eat the forbidden fruit promising her that, 'Ye shall be as gods, knowing good and evil.'

So Eve, 'Did eat, and gave also unto her husband with her; and he did eat. Then their eyes were opened, their innocence lost, they sewed fig leaves together and made themselves aprons with which they covered their pudenda (Latin, pudenda membra - parts to be ashamed of).'

Unleashed in one fell swoop were the driving forces of religion; morality; guilt, lust, and knowledge of what is right and what is wrong in the eyes of the Church. The Christian Church throughout the Middle Ages was all-powerful. The 'thou shalt not' words of the Commandments, the words of Jesus and the edicts of saints and theologians formed the rules of life; obedience to them determined one's fate in the Hereafter. There has never been a more powerful weapon than the threat of eternal damnation in the fires of hell.

LONG BEFORE THE MIDDLE AGES THERE WERE CONVENTIONS of civilised behaviour, such as those which governed the societies of Ancient Egypt,

Greece, and the Roman Empire. Although the Romans had a liberal attitude to, and took delight in, sexual pastimes, they observed an etiquette which saw performances by couples in the open, on a park bench or in full view on a boat, as vulgar.

The violent eruption of Mount Vesuvius in 79AD resulted in the Roman cities of Pompeii and Herculaneum being almost instantaneously covered in a layer of searing pyroclastic ash and pumice up to six metres deep. The inhabitants died rapidly of thermal shock in an all-enveloping volcanic cloud at a temperature of 500°C. The sheer speed of the disaster had an effect like freezing a film frame. Excavations revealed beautiful frescoes and mosaics and excavation of houses showed how the Romans led their daily lives, stored their food, did their cooking, and other humdrum aspects of Roman life. Some houses boasted a cubiculum (Latin, from cubare - to lie down), a separate room, where couples could indulge in private when taken by a sudden fancy. Excavations also revealed that the Romans regarded the erect penis as talismanic; plaster models of the priapic member, in startling profile, decorated the walls of streets and houses, some were more than simply decorative, they pointed towards the nearest brothel.

The word fornication, meaning sex between unmarried couples, had its origin in ancient Rome. A fornix (Latin, from fornix - originally, a vaulted chamber, later, a brothel) was originally a secluded room in the Roman amphitheatre; a tier of fornices encircled the highest level of the auditorium. Couples of different or the same sexes could take their pleasures, in private, in the intervals between gladiatorial bouts or the feeding of lions with undesirables, such as serious criminals and Christians.

Christianity was scarcely visible in first century Rome, Judaism was much more noticeable. Jews were tolerated; they had lived an independent existence under Roman law since 200BC. In Palestine, the Jewish persecution of

Christians caused converts to Christianity to flee to various parts of the Roman Empire. At that time Rome, the nerve centre of the known world, attracted most immigrants. For that reason it also attracted many of the Apostles, including Peter and Paul, the latter had been specifically commanded to take the message of Christ to the Gentiles.

The great fire of Rome in 64AD lasted six days and nights. Nero (37-68AD, Emperor 54-68AD) heard rumours that Rome's citizens blamed him for it, saying that he had caused the fire for his own amusement or alternatively, that he wanted to clear an area in which to build a new palace. The Roman historian, Tacitus, recorded that to deflect the accusation Nero fingered Christian communities living close to where the fire began, and declared, 'All Christians are evil, their leader was a criminal. Rome arrested him, tried him, found him guilty and executed him.'

On Nero's command hundreds of Christians were rounded up and tortured to death. The general hostility towards Christians lasted more than three centuries during which time thousands of Christians were martyred. The Romans regarded Christianity with suspicion, to them it was not a proper religion but some sort of cannibalistic superstition… in their ceremonies they consumed the body of Christ and because they called each other Brother and Sister it was assumed that incest was rife.

Nero was not an endearing character; fortunately at the age of thirty-one he committed suicide. Had he lived a normal span heaven alone knows what further mischief he might have wrought. Not only was he responsible for the wholesale slaughter of Christians, his domestic life was chaotic; he killed his mother in 55AD, his first wife in 62AD and his second wife when, allegedly, he kicked her in the belly when she was heavily pregnant.

A successor to Nero, Domitian (Emperor 89-96AD), encouraged even greater cruelty; he mounted public spectacles to entertain the citizenry. He had Christian families brutally killed by lions or gladiators in 'sporting' contests in the arenas of amphitheatres. Over the first three centuries of the Middle Ages the persecution of Christians gained momentum and spread throughout the Roman Empire. The Romans avowed that the Christians had only themselves to blame; they refused to conform to Roman standards, they would not accept the divine status of the Emperor, and they refused to worship the Gods of Rome.

It was under Emperor Diocletian (245-311AD) that the last, largest, and bloodiest official persecution occurred. One morning, at a meeting of the Senate, a senator told him that he had received a message from the Gods which told him that all Christians should be slaughtered. Diocletian consulted the Oracle of Apollo, for himself. The Oracle confirmed that the advice was indeed genuine and The Great Diocletian Persecution was launched with mass executions of Christians at the beginning of 303AD.

Diocletian was a capable economist and during his reign (284-305AD) succeeded in returning Rome to such a sound financial footing that the ailing empire was able to totter along for another century. Diocletian retired at the age of fifty-eight because of ill health. Competing for his throne were two junior Caesars, Maximine and Constantine. Fortunately, for Christianity, Constantine was appointed the ruler of most of the Roman Empire.

Maximine ruled over Italy and North Africa and when he retired his son, Maxentius, took over. Maxentius was popular; like politicians down the ages he gained support by promising to reduce taxes. He led two unsuccessful uprisings in attempting to usurp Constantine who became the overriding focus of his hatred, always referring to him as 'that son of a harlot.'

DURING THE REIGN OF EMPEROR CONSTANTINE (306-337AD) CHRISTIANITY WAS ACCEPTED and gained so much popularity that it became the preferred religion. Two factors brought about the change. The first, Constantine's mother, Helena, was a devout Christian and influenced her son to convert. Helena was of humble origin, said to be a barmaid when she met Constantine's father, Constantius, a general in the Roman army. When Helena was eighty she made a pilgrimage to the Holy Land and returned to Rome with relics of the True Cross, for this, centuries later, she was canonized as Saint Helena of Constantinople.

Incidentally, on 25 May 1502, an isolated island in the middle of the vast Atlantic Ocean was spotted by a Portuguese explorer and because it was St Helena of Constantinople's birthday, the explorer named the island for her.

The second factor, and crucial to the rapidity of the emergence of Christianity, was that Constantine experienced two powerful messages the night before doing battle with Maxentius. The first message arrived in the evening sky with the appearance of a dazzling light which formed the words, 'in hoc signo vinces' (with this sign you will conquer). The second message arrived during the night in the form of a dream in which Constantine was visited by a vision of Christ. The vision guaranteed victory if his soldiers marked Christ's heavenly sign, the Chi-Rho, a P with a cross on the stem, on their shields. Each soldier made the mark and the battle was won, even though Constantine's army was at least a third smaller than that of Maxentius.

The battle took place at the end of 312AD near the Milvian Bridge, which stands to this day and spans the Tiber to the north of Rome. Wounded and weighed down by his armour Maxentius fell into the river and drowned. Next day his corpse was found, retrieved, stripped of its armour and beheaded. The separated head and body were displayed in Rome and then exhibited all over the empire to demonstrate to Maxentius's followers that he was indeed dead, and that he had suffered the fate in store for all those who dared to take arms against Emperor Constantine.

The Romans worshipped many gods; Jupiter, Juno, Mars, Apollo, Diana, Mithras, and scores of local deities. To the Romans, in general, Christianity did not rate highly, it was merely an obscure branch of Judaism but that changed dramatically with the Edict of Milan (313AD) in which Constantine decreed full tolerance for Christianity, and all religions. From then on the increasing dominance of the Christian Church and repeated meetings of councils at the highest level led to the codification of all forms of behaviour, including sexual, acceptable to the Church.

In the last hundred years of its existence the Roman Empire was in turmoil. It is likely that Constantine had hoped to exert a unifying force by declaring his Christianity and decreeing tolerance for all religions. Backing every horse in the race he continued to patronise the pantheon of Roman gods, including Mithras. However, not long before he died Constantine was baptised and thus he placed, for all time, the imperial seal of approval on Christianity.

Rome did not fall overnight; it crumbled over the fourth and fifth centuries. Various Germanic tribes attacked Rome but the year 410AD saw the biggest calamity when on 24 August the city was sacked by a Gothic army led by Alaric. The government was evacuated to Byzantium, which by then had been renamed Constantinople in the Emperor's honour. The collapse of Rome left the city and known world in chaos with only one stable organisation in the midst of a political and cultural morass... the burgeoning Christian Church. A new era was dawning, the Middle Ages, and it would last a thousand years.

ROME BECAME THE HEADQUARTERS OF CHRISTIANITY, it was a natural choice. By the end of the fourth century Rome had a sizeable population of

Christians and the major Apostles, Peter and Paul, had been martyred there. Born a Roman citizen, St Paul had visited Rome on two occasions, each for long periods. St Peter had spent twenty years in Rome and became the Bishop of Rome, effectively the first Pope. His public martyrdom took place three months after Nero burned Rome and was included as a grand spectacle in the entertainment programme of Christian persecutions. St Peter was crucified, upside-down at his own request, but St Paul, because he was a citizen of Rome, could not be crucified, he was beheaded.

The attitude of the Christian Church to sex, marriage, women, and sin evolved from the very beginnings of the religion. By the early Middle Ages, and following many conferences and councils of the elders, the Church's attitude to every aspect of life on earth and in the hereafter was formulated. The Christian Church followed the teachings of St Paul on women: 'They were created second, sinned first and should keep silence.'

He took this teaching further when he stressed that women must be silent in church: 'Let your women keep silence in the church: for it is not permitted unto them to speak but they are commanded to be under obedience, as also saith, "the law."'

That couldn't be much clearer but to be quite sure Saint Paul added, '… for it is a shame for women to speak in the church.'

St Paul's teachings continued throughout medieval Europe and linger to this day for the more conservative Christian Churches. It is only in the last century and a half that feminist movements and sophisticated thinking have had any liberating effects on attitudes to women in general and their place in the Anglican and Nonconformist communities.

As far as sex was concerned St Paul believed that celibacy and chastity were superior to marriage because they eliminated emotions which would interfere with religious obligations. St Paul recognised human frailty and accepted marriage as a necessary sacrament, declaring it blessed by God and sanctified by Christ: 'But if they cannot contain, let them marry: for it is better to marry than to burn.'

The Church regarded matrimony as a concession to human weakness, as a necessity for the procreation of children and to provide lifelong companionship. Saint Jerome (347-420AD) had some startling things to say about marriage, celibacy, human love and above all his unbound admiration for virginity. Perhaps St Jerome is best known for his translation of the bible into Latin, the Vulgate Bible. He was also the Abbot who, when a lion limped into his monastery scattering fellow clerics like hens before a fox, picked up the lion's sore paw and removed a thorn from it with a pair of golden tweezers.

St Jerome said he 'Did not disparage marriage when I set virginity before it ... marriage is honoured when it is placed next to virginity ... and so I practise marriage because it brings forth virginity – thus do I pluck a rose from thorns, the gold from the earth, the pearl from the shell.'

If these concepts are difficult to understand, he said something even more confusing: 'omnis ardentior amatori propriae uxoris adulterer est,' – passionate love by a man of his own wife is adultery.

In other words, if a man is head-over-heels in love with his wife, he is in a state of permanent sin. St Jerome recounted that when inadvertently (but only) in his imagination he found himself watching dancing Roman maidens and felt the call of the flesh, he could only purge himself by weeks of fasting. His pronouncement, 'Whosoever looketh on a woman, to lust after her, hath committed adultery already in his heart.' would resonate with any normal male, and like the Rev MacMaking's threats to me, implant everlasting guilt.

IN THEIR ATTITUDES TO WOMEN CHRISTIAN THEOLOGIANS and saints spoke their minds frankly, but their teachings were mild compared with the early teachings of Islam. The legend of The Garden of Eden and The Fall of Eve is as seminal in Islam as it was to Christians in the Middle Ages. More than four centuries after the death of the Prophet Mohammed, Imam al Ghazali (1058-1111), a respected Islamic teacher of his time, wrote in his 'Counsel for Kings' that for Eve's disobedience the Almighty God had decreed eighteen punishments for women. The first three were menstruation, pregnancy, and childbirth. Next, a woman was liable to divorce on her husband's say-so but she was not able to initiate divorce herself. Al Ghazali also stated that it is lawful for men to have four wives but women can have only one husband. Further that she must stay secluded in the house with her head covered and that she must not go out of the house unless accompanied.

The Imam went on to declare that in law women are disqualified from being rulers and judges and that the testimony of two women has to be weighed against that of one man. In religious observance, men could take part in Friday prayers, feast day prayers and funeral prayers but women could not. Al Ghazali also wrote that Merit has a thousand components, only one of which is attributable to women… while nine hundred and ninety nine are attributable to men. In his Counsel he included strictures on women remarrying after divorce or the death of their husbands. Finally, those women who had been profligate in life would be punished more harshly than men on the day of resurrection.

After all the pronouncements by Christian saints it is no wonder that it took almost two millennia for women to even get the vote in England. In Islam the present position is much as Al Ghazali taught; historically Islam lags six hundred years behind Christianity. One cannot too often repeat the observation that it was men who made these declarations concerning women, and that those men were the wise men, the saints, the hakims, the imams, and the sages of the major religions.

IN MEDIEVAL CHRISTIANITY, SEXUAL INTERCOURSE was unclean and shameful. The conception of Jesus was, however, not through a shameful act, his conception was through the Holy Spirit entering the womb of the Virgin Mary... who was herself sin free and in a state of permanent grace. Mary had been immaculately conceived of Anne, wife of Joachim, and therefore was, herself, without original sin.

Saint Augustine (354-436) maintained that Mary, conceived as a virgin, lived as a virgin, gave birth as a virgin, and died a virgin. His prayer, 'Lord, give me chastity, but not yet,' is often quoted in an almost humorous vein, but the quotation is usually made out of context. St Augustine uttered his prayer long before he converted to Christianity, at a time when he was still living a wild youth. In his teachings St Augustine declared that women were intellectually and morally inferior to men. To support this opinion he cited the action of the Serpent; that it was Eve the Serpent approached because he knew that she was a soft touch, unintelligent and lacking self-control.

The Church had such a hold on the affairs of men during the Middle Ages that the only way of pursuing a career in law, civil administration or academia, was by first entering the priesthood. That was tolerable until the fifteenth century when by papal decree bishops and priests were banned from marrying and commanded to live celibate and continent lives.

Marriage conferred the right to sexual intercourse. Sexual intercourse was legitimate only within marriage. Marriage was a concession to human weakness; it was solely for the purpose of procreation. Intercourse performed without reproduction in mind was sinful, to take pleasure in the act made it doubly so.

Recognising that intercourse was an inevitable part of marriage various authorities sought to regulate its frequency. Before Christianity came on the scene a Greek statesman, Solon (638-558BC), the founder of Athenian democracy and a renowned sage was so concerned by the decline in morals in Athens that he declared that intercourse three times a month was quite enough. The Jewish Mishnah (the law in writing, previously having been transmitted by word-of-mouth) stated that the frequency of intercourse should be: every day for the unemployed, twice a week for labourers and donkey drivers, once a month for camel drivers and for sailors, once every six months.

Early Christian theologians also elaborated exact rules for the frequency of intercourse for married couples. Abstention on Thursdays in memory of Christ's arrest; abstention on Fridays, in memory of his death; abstention on Saturdays, in honour of the Virgin Mary and abstention on Sundays, in honour of the Resurrection. There remained Mondays, Tuesdays, and Wednesdays, but these were not necessarily days of sexual licence because abstention was recommended during the forty days of Lent, during Easter, Pentecost, Christmas, and on Saints' days. This censorious attitude to intercourse persists to modern times. In 1978 the Archbishop of Canterbury ordered that the two hundred bishops attending the Lambeth Conference should be housed apart from their wives for the three week's duration of the meeting.

Human nature being what it is there were plenty of transgressors. The Church dealt with transgressions by awarding punishments, which were called penances. Spiritually cleansed by carrying out the penances, and on condition that they sinned no more, the Church could permit entry into paradise.

The Church held authority not only over the frequency of the sexual act, it also determined the one and only position permitted during the act. Later called 'The Missionary Position,' the man would be superior with the woman lying supine and passive beneath him. It was the only form of copulation the Church allowed; other postures were likened to animal behaviour. And just as variations from standard intercourse were not countenanced, other means of sexual gratification were forbidden; solitary and mutual masturbation, homosexual sex, use of dildos by nuns, oral sex, anal sex, pederasty, coitus interruptus, and even male nocturnal emissions, all attracted the Church's attention, disapprobation, and punishment.. St Augustine declared a man's spontaneous erection as sinful, but added that it did not attract punishment because it was involuntary.

DIFFICULTIES WERE EXPERIENCED IN THE ROMAN ARMY in the early days of Christianity. Soldiers, the defenders of the Empire and the guardians of law and order, were traditionally worshippers of Mithras. When they converted to Christianity at Constantine's command, Roman soldiers continued to practise homosexuality and pederasty, both of which were a normal part of what was an exclusively male preserve, the cult of Mithraism.

There was no ambivalence in Christian teaching in the matter of homosexuality. St Thomas Aquinas (1225-1274) argued that because the Creator had designed the sexual organs for reproduction, and reproduction only, it was a sin to use them in any way which did not encompass the possibility of conception. He further declared that God's destruction of Sodom and Gomorrah gave a clear message condemning homosexual behaviour.

Recognising that monastic life could give rise to temptation, monks were forbidden to share the same bed. Dormitories of nuns were to be lit by a lamp throughout the night and in fear of baths arousing auto-erotic feelings, nuns in strict orders were commanded to wear a vest while performing their ablutions.

In the sixth century it was taught that homosexuality and blasphemy gave rise to divine punishment in the form of famines, earthquakes, and pestilence. The Emperor Justinian shared this view and shortly after he declared his support he was proved correct by the onset of the Great Plague of 541AD which wiped out a third of the population of Constantinople. It is a matter for speculation that Justinian himself had the plague, but recovered.

In some quarters this punitive belief persists into the 21st century. Within days of the event assorted zealous evangelicals announced that the Pacific tsunami in December 2004 was God's judgement on the world's homosexuality. Exactly three years later a British theologian, the Bishop of Carlisle, pronounced in December 2007 that extensive flooding in the north of England was due to the permissive attitude to homosexuality in that region. Although Carlisle is not generally known as a hotbed of gay behaviour it was there that the worst floods occurred. Curiously, trendy homes of homosexuality, London and Brighton for example, escaped inundation.

To unify the penalties for transgressors throughout the Christian world the Roman Church hierarchy enacted a law which dictated a comprehensive list of punishments. These were in the form of penances and some were extreme. At the end of the seventh century one of the many councils of Toledo, describing sodomy as being prevalent in Spain, ruled that 'if any one of those males who commit this vile practice against nature with other males is a bishop, a priest or a deacon, he shall be degraded from the dignity of his order, and shall remain in perpetual exile, struck down by damnation.'

A hundred lashes, a shaven head, and banishment were standard punishments imposed by the Church on laymen, later castration was added.

Manuals to unify penances awarded in confessionals were issued to priests in the early Middle Ages. The severity of the penance varied according to the customs of the time and the degree of the offence. Simple kissing between same sexes under the age of twenty merited six fasts. Habitual mutual masturbation between males over the age of twenty was punished by penance for a year. Doing penance involved public confession of the sin, fasting for specified periods on bread and water, and for a year or more standing at the door of the church before services and professing contrition. Penitents, guilty of serious offences were banished to far countries where in groups they would go on tour dressed in sackcloth, doused in ashes and publicly scourging themselves – and each other.

The centuries following the end of the first millennium saw changes in the attitudes of the Church and mankind towards women; an age of churlishness gave way to an age of chivalry. Women were no better off financially, legally, or physically, and the precepts of Saints Augustine, Paul and Thomas Aquinas still held sway, but men's ideas of womankind had improved beyond measure. Men turned women into ladies, who then became symbols of innocence and virtue. It was the two centuries of the Crusades which brought about the change. The Crusades were the military campaigns fought by the Christians of Europe between the eleventh and thirteenth centuries to regain the holy lands the Muslims had conquered, and in particular, the holy city of Jerusalem.

Men's attitudes to women underwent more changes in the centuries of the Crusades than in the thousand years before. The new emphasis was more on woman's innate virtue and morality than stressing her second rate status. Putting their ladies on pedestals, however, gave rise to feelings of insecurity among men, feelings exacerbated by the prospect of being away for years fighting holy wars.

WHAT COULD BE DONE? MEN COULD LOCK AWAY THEIR MONEY and treasures; why not lock up their women? The solution was the chastity belt; developed in Italy it was called The Florentine Girdle. It was made as a metal frame which surrounded the upper thighs and had a metal strut-like piece extending from the pubes in front to the upper part of the cleft between the buttocks behind. There were two apertures for waste elimination, which equally prevented penetration. The apparatus was locked over the hips and the husband held the key.

It has to be said that there is debate as to whether chastity belts did actually exist at the time of the Crusades. And it would seem self-evident that locksmiths could easily fashion keys for the locks of such crude contraptions. Chastity belts exist today, they are not expensive and can be bought through the Internet; they are used as anti-rape devices or, puzzlingly, in some form of sex play.

In December 2003 a security alarm at Athens airport was triggered by a metal chastity belt, the flustered passenger explained that her husband had forced her to wear it whilst on holiday in Greece. The understanding and sympathetic captain of the aircraft allowed her to continue her journey.

Times have changed since the pronouncements of the many medieval Councils of Toledo to protect souls from the ravages of all forms of sexual misbehaviour. A councilwoman in another Toledo, in Ohio, in the United States of America, in December 2012 announced her support for gay marriage on the basis that – 'It will increase tourism.'

2. SEX – FROM GOOD QUEEN BESS TO PRINCE PRINNY

WAS THE VIRGIN QUEEN A MAN? There is a theory that the first Queen Elizabeth, affectionately known as Good Queen Bess, was genetically a man and that was because she was an example of the Testicular Feminization Syndrome, a rare congenital disorder which was subsequently renamed, the Androgen Insensitivity Syndrome (AIS).

AIS results when the subject has the chromosomal XY makeup of a male – not the XX of a female – yet outwardly appears to be a woman... and often a beautiful woman. The fault lies in the sexual development of the foetus. Early in its life the embryo has primitive gonads, the default setting of which is that they are destined to become ovaries and the child will therefore be female.

If, however, the Y chromosome is present in the genetic makeup, at six weeks after conception, a gene on the Y chromosome directs the development of the ovaries to become testes. The testes produce male sex hormones, androgens, and thereafter normal foetal development is masculine.

Rarely the foetal sex tissues do not respond to the influence of androgens and their development is deranged. A proper penis and other male characteristics do not appear. Individuals with AIS have testicles which do not descend from whence they originate in the abdomen. The penis is rudimentary and may appear like a clitoris. The empty scrotum at birth can look like female external genitalia with an aperture of varying depth resembling a vaginal entrance. At puberty the development of secondary sexual characteristics, including breast growth, are female.

If the theory about her gender is correct when Queen Elizabeth, in her famous speech rallying the army at Tilbury, declaimed, 'I know I have the body of a weak and feeble woman but I have the heart and stomach of a king.' she may have spoken the literal truth. Maybe Good Queen Bess had other kingly anatomical attributes, a pair of testicles, hidden inside her abdomen.

The first Queen Elizabeth had many male characteristics; in her youth she was extremely athletic, she had an aggressive personality, she remained unmarried, and her gloves showed her fourth (ring) fingers to be longer than her index fingers. Other, possibly male, attributes were that she swore like a trooper, picked her teeth with a golden toothpick, and took delight in coarse jokes. For what it's worth, an epigram surfaced in the hoi polloi a few years after Elizabeth's successor, James I (who was known to more than favour handsome male courtiers) ascended the throne: 'She was King Elizabeth and now we have Queen James.'

Good Queen Bess, nevertheless, had many men friends, the closest of which was Robert Dudley, the first Earl of Leicester; she called him her, 'Sweet Robin.' The relationship could not bloom because he was already married. Surprisingly, Sweet Robin's young wife, Amy, died after accidentally falling down a flight of stairs. Rumours abounded that Dudley had engineered the accident. The scandal was so credible that Elizabeth declared that marriage with Sweet Robin could never take place.

Although court chatter whispered that the Earl of Leicester came within a codpiece of marrying Bess it also whispered that she 'had a membrane so strong that it made her incapable of men.' That would further support the notion of her having the androgen insensitivity syndrome; in which case she would merely have a short canal representing a rudimentary vagina.

Could the origin of the rumour that she was incapable of men have its basis in one of her court physicians letting it slip? It seems more than likely that at some time in her early life she had suspicions that she couldn't bear children. For this she might have sought medical advice which would almost certainly have involved a physical examination. Perhaps her anatomical abnormality was leaked, but whatever the reason; Elizabeth never married and referred to herself as, 'The Virgin Queen' throughout her reign.

She had other close men friends; Sir Philip Sydney, Sir Christopher Hatton, and of course the most celebrated – Sir Walter Raleigh. That friendship was said to have begun on a rainy day when he was out walking with the Queen and her entourage. They came across a muddy puddle, promptly Sir Walter gallantly swept off his cloak and laid it across the puddle so that Her Majesty could step on it and not dirty her new fine-leather shoes. For many years, even though Raleigh spoke like a Devon yokel, he was her favourite at court.

But there is no proof that Elizabeth ever had full sexual relations with a man. As the Queen of England she would have been under surveillance for twenty four hours a day and seven days a week. Moreover, she usually slept with one or two Ladies of the Chamber in her bed; Queen Bess feared the dark.

Elizabeth died on 24 March 1603, she was nearly seventy. It was said that she died of blood poisoning, but poisoning with what? Her death did not have the turbulence associated with the usual cause of blood poisoning, a severe infection leading to septicaemia; it was a quiet passing, over a few days. Was she poisoned by her makeup? Some have implicated the thick white paste she used to cover the facial scars left by the severe attack of smallpox she had survived in 1562 when she was twenty-nine years old.

The makeup she used was called Ceruse. It was a mixture of white lead and vinegar. Such paste would cause skin ulceration which would enhance the absorption of lead and as the ulceration progressed she would need to apply thicker and thicker layers. Yet another theory is that the paste which killed Elizabeth contained arsenic. The most plausible theory, however, is that she simply died of old age – sixty-nine was old for those days.

It will never be known whether in fact she had the androgen insensitivity syndrome. She had decreed that her body should not be opened after death; there would be no post-mortem examination. Her body was prepared for interment exclusively by her ladies-in-waiting.

OVER SEVENTEEN YEARS AFTER GOOD QUEEN BESS DIED, the Mayflower, a cargo ship long past its prime, sailed from the English port of Plymouth bound for the New World, three thousand miles away. The Mayflower set sail on 6 September 1620 and carried a hundred and two Puritans. Seventy-three men and twenty-nine women (including eighteen married couples) were cramped together in abysmally low-ceilinged quarters on a floor space which in total amounted to the area of a tennis court; each person was limited to a space the size of an adult coffin.

During the voyage there were two deaths and one birth. One of the dead was a sailor who died before the Mayflower had reached halfway across the Atlantic; the cause of his death is not recorded but was probably acute

appendicitis. To the pilgrims it was an act of Providence –
they described him as 'mean spirited' – soon after the
Mayflower had left the sheltered waters of Plymouth
Sound he took great delight in taunting passengers who
were seasick.

Members of Christian churches which had separated
from the Church of Rome were collectively called
Protestants, and while the Puritans on the Mayflower were
Protestants, they were also fleeing the strictures of the
Anglican Church. They had no respect for the English
established church which they looked upon as a product of
political struggle and man-made doctrine. To them it had
not distanced itself far enough from the Church of Rome.
Total Papal servitude, the command of clerical celibacy
and vows of continence were principles which
Nonconformists vehemently opposed.

The Mayflower came in sight of land on 9 November
1620. The Puritans formed the Plymouth Colony in what
is now Plymouth, Massachusetts. William Bradford, who
was one of the Puritans on the Mayflower, was the first to
call them The Pilgrim Fathers. About half of the colonists
died, many from scurvy, in the first winter. Of the eighteen
wives, thirteen succumbed.

For some years men seriously outnumbered women.
Inevitably this gave rise to problems caused by sexual
frustration; an extreme example was that of a teenage
servant, Thomas Granger. He was found guilty of having
carnal knowledge of a mare, a cow, two goats, five sheep,
two calves, and a turkey. Punishment was extreme, first the
hapless animals were lined up and shot in front of him…
and then he was hanged.

The morality of the Puritans was destined to affect
American future cultural attitudes. It produced a mental
state which to some extent resembled that of the
Victorians in England some two centuries later. Whilst
maintaining a biblical subservience to their husbands in
sexual matters, women developed control of their menfolk

by means of virtue and piety. The concept of a God-fearing, Bible-loving family became the cornerstone of American social development.

In succeeding decades the Pilgrim Fathers were followed by immigrants who were, like them, Protestant Nonconformists; Quakers, Baptists, Swedish, Finnish, and German Lutherans. Later, as the New World's attraction grew as a sanctuary from problems at home not only Nonconformists but Anglicans, Roman Catholics, Quakers, and Jews poured in from Europe and in particular, Roman Catholics from Ireland, and were all accepted as equals by the welcoming arms of the United States of America.

The original Puritans were dour and colourless people. Premarital sex was strictly taboo but intramarital sex was encouraged and enthusiastically enjoyed. In those days of gross imbalance in the sex ratio bestiality was a capital offence, but even so was a recurring problem. A one-eyed servant, George Spencer, who had many times been on the wrong side of the law, was arrested when a sow dropped a one-eyed piglet in her litter. The sow was admitted as a witness by the examining magistrate. Spencer was found guilty and hanged.

Meanwhile in Europe religious upheavals in the sixteenth and seventeenth centuries were changing the fabric of a society which had become overly strait-laced. As usual the Church of Rome proceeded on its authoritarian way, it reinforced the attitude that virginity was a more blessed state than marriage and that celibacy of its ordained clergy was compulsory. The Wars of Religion, essentially Catholic versus Protestant, were pursued between various European countries for more than a century.

THE AGE OF ENLIGHTENMENT BEGAN in the middle of the seventeenth century and ushered in a sea change in intellectual, cultural and scientific thinking. By the middle of the eighteenth century the sexual mores of England and Europe had undergone a revolution – a rupture more dramatic than that declared two centuries later by the poet Philip Larkin who said, 'sexual intercourse began in 1963', referring to the sexual liberation of women by the contraceptive pill.

Dr Samuel Johnson (1709-1784), lover of London, lexicographer, fount of bons mots and a Tory High Anglican, said among his hundreds of quotable aphorisms: 'Every man should regulate his actions according to his own conscience.'

Johnson's advice was eagerly snapped up by his good friend and biographer, James Boswell (1740-1795), who had already suffered nineteen attacks of the clap (gonorrhoea) before he first met Dr Johnson in a London bookshop on 16 May 1763.

Boswell particularly enjoyed what he called 'sixpenny knee-tremblers' in St James's Park. Generously he shared his pleasure by recounting episodes of his favourite pastime in his journal. On Tuesday 10 May 1763, he wrote: 'At the bottom of the Haymarket I picked up a strong, jolly young damsel and taking her under the arm I conducted her to Westminster Bridge, and there in armour complete did I engage her upon this noble edifice. The whim of doing so there with the Thames rolling below amused me much.'

On another occasion Boswell wrote that he had enjoyed a dalliance with seventeen year old Alice Briggs in the back garden of the official residence of the Prime Minister, 10 Downing Street. Hopefully the Tory Prime Minister, Lord North, was so busy with affairs of state, (losing Britain's American colonies) that he didn't observe the goings-on in the middle of the hydrangeas.

The 'armour complete' he wore was a condom. Boswell, a man of experience and judgement was of the opinion that the best condoms in London were available in Leicester Square at an inn called The Sign of the Rising

Sun. They were hand made by a Mrs Phillips, her best quality were called Baudriches Superfine. The meaning of baudriche is unclear; it could simply be 'a balloon.' Mrs Phillips finest were made of two layers of sheep intestine gummed together, perfumed and fashioned on glass moulds. Cheaper condoms were available - made of high quality fine linen, they had to be dipped in water immediately before use; Boswell found the Hyde Park Canal convenient. They had the advantage of being reusable and Boswell would take his, in batches, to Jenny's condom laundry in St Martin's Lane.

Condoms were secured by being tied with a ribbon at the base. Gentlemen could have the ribbon coloured as they pleased. Mrs Phillips would oblige with regimental colours, the brilliant red and yellow of the governing body of cricket, the Marylebone Cricket Club, the pink and green of the Garrick Club, or any colours a dandy might fancy.

When Boswell wasn't writing, or taking a dish of tea with Dr Johnson (who averaged fourteen dishes a day), his life was one of a succession of sexual adventures punctuated by spells of treatment for repeated infections with the clap. The clap causes a copious penile discharge of pus, a sign commonly known as the gleet. A medical student story has it that a certain Lord So-and-So presented himself to a London, Harley-Street doctor, a clap specialist, complaining, 'I have a cold in my John Thomas.'

Whereupon the physician took out his fob watch, looked at the offending member, with a bead of pus hanging at the urethral meatus – the tip, and said,

'A cold, Milord? If it doesn't sneeze in one minute you've got the clap.'

Before the advent of antibiotics the treatment of the clap was highly unsatisfactory. Recurrent infections led to the formation of strictures in the urethra of the penis. Strictures are scars produced by inflammation. The diameter of the penile urethra (the channel through which urine flows) becomes so narrowed that to pass urine, straining with enormous effort was necessary. I have recounted elsewhere (*DOCTOR LARK – the benefits of a medical education*) how I encountered highly-polished brass 'straining bars' at shoulder-height above the men's urinals when I was a member of the Penang Club in Malaysia. They were conveniently placed to assist planters who had acquired urethral strictures as a result of dallying with lady rubber tree tappers.

The only remedy for strictures then was to pass what are called 'sounds' (curved metal rods) of increasing diameter down the urethra to force open the scarred and narrowed segments. Boswell loathed this treatment. The pain and embarrassment must have made his toes curl; nowadays doctors squeeze local anaesthetic jelly into a man's urethra before performing procedures involving the passage of instruments. As it happened an acute inability to pass urine was to finish off Boswell. In 1795 after a long dinner with the bibulous members of the Literary Club of London he was carried home unable to pass a drop; he died a few days later.

It is a sobering thought that there is now clear evidence that strains of the bacterium which causes gonorrhoea, the gonococcus (Neisseria gonorrhoeae), have become resistant to the antibiotics most often used in its treatment; in time it may become resistant to all antibiotics. With antibiotic-resistant gonorrhoea the bad old days of urethral strictures will return. Whole hospital outpatient clinic sessions will then be relegated to junior doctors passing sounds; a pastime which neither patients nor doctors enjoy.

If you look at the gonococcus through a microscope it doesn't look so nasty. In the usual Gram-stained pus smears it looks like a pair of red kidney beans nestling quietly inside a white blood cell… but its looks belie its nature. It can cause severe inflammation of the rectum leading to rectal strictures and it can cause awful complications by infecting the joints, the eyes, the heart, and the nervous system.

WHILE JAMES BOSWELL WAS ENJOYING HIS LARKS IN THE PARK in London a certain Donatien Alphonse François de Sade was larking about on the other side of the English Channel, but in strikingly different ways. His youth had been blighted by an uncle who had introduced him to group sex including both men and women; this was at the age of six, at about the same age his nurse thrashed him until he enjoyed it.

As a young man he paid for adventures with groups of prostitutes. Sometimes he gave them an aphrodisiac powder which contained cantharidin, commonly known as Spanish fly. The powder is made by pounding together dried beetles of a species frequently found in Spain and which secrete the intensely irritant cantharidin. Usually the beetle powder was mixed with wine and taken by mouth. Cantharidin owes its aphrodisiac property to causing an intense irritation of the genitalia. It is excreted in the urine via the kidneys.

But Spanish fly is dangerous; a high dose destroys kidney tissue and quickly leads to death from renal failure. I well remember the Case of Lethal Coconut Icing Poisoning from my medical student days. An office Lothario, working in Euston Road, close to my teaching hospital, gave a couple of typist girls coconut icing laced with Spanish fly. The girls were admitted in extreme distress caused by the intense irritation of their bladders and urethras. They rapidly went into renal failure, one died in fifteen hours and the other a day later; those were the days before kidney dialysis. In my mind's eye I can still see, vividly, the pathologist displaying the startlingly severe, haemorrhagic bladder inflammation.

The Marquis de Sade, however, knew his toxicology and was careful, as far as we know he never gave a lethal dose. He had other amusing pastimes. On occasion he would pay to watch a group of naked prostitutes, with peacock feathers projecting from their fundamental orifices, prancing around a room on their hands and knees, while at other times, he employed them to thrash him with a red-hot cat o'nine tails. In addition to his masochistic leaning he relished giving physical pain, and so much did his reputation for this pastime grow that he gave his name to the perverted pleasure obtained from inflicting pain, sadism.

His carryings-on frequently got him into trouble; although well paid some ladies did not enjoy pain the way he did and even though he was of the lesser French nobility, his title, the Marquis de Sade, could not protect him from spending in all thirty-two of his seventy-four years incarcerated, either in jail or in a lunatic asylum. He was in the Bastille prison up to a few days before the first day of the Revolution on 14 July 1789. On 2 July he repeatedly shouted from a window to the crowd outside, 'Help! Help! They are killing prisoners in here!'

He was swiftly transferred to an insane asylum at Charenton, near Paris. He was released in 1790, and although he was the prime exemplar of sadism he admitted that he found the Revolution's Reign of Terror excessively cruel.

The Marquis de Sade was elected as a delegate to the National Council (the first French Assembly) in 1792 and served for three years. How that came about is not known and it is bizarre that a man so recently an inpatient in a lunatic asylum could have been elected to the Revolutionary Government, but those were strange times in France. In present day France your average Frenchman would think it a credible explanation for the current political state of his country.

The Marquis didn't fritter away his time when confined or imprisoned. He wrote books, one with the engaging title, One Hundred and Twenty Days of Sodom. He wrote plays which were staged with a cast drawn from his fellow prisoners, asylum inmates or staff. Performances were stopped when the content became particularly outrageous and once he so offended the governor of a jail that he was thrown into solitary confinement without pen or paper.

When he died at the age of seventy-four he had spent the last thirteen years of his life in the Charenton asylum in which he had been incarcerated for a year at the time of the French Revolution. Fortunately for him the asylum was run by a kindly religious order, the Brothers of Charity, under an enlightened senior cleric, the Abbé de Coulmier. The Marquis de Sade's final fling involved Madeleine Leclerc, a daughter of one of the asylum guardians. She was a mere girl, thirteen years old at the start of their affair. He recorded the tally of his encounters with Madeleine in his journal; they had their ultimate tryst four days before he died in his sleep.

JAMES GRAHAM (1745-1794) STUDIED MEDICINE AT EDINBURGH UNIVERSITY but left without taking a degree. Nevertheless he was able to set himself up as an apothecary and after practising for a short while in the county of Yorkshire in the north of England, and marrying, he went to the United States of America. There, without further training, he became a travelling specialist in diseases of the eyes and ears. In Philadelphia he was invited to observe the marvellously curative properties of electricity. Impressed by its possibilities he hotfooted it back to London where he established what he called his 'medico-magnetico-musico-electrico treatment centre.'

In May 1780 he opened The Temple of Health in the Adelphi. Treatments advertised included musical therapy, pneumatic chemistry, and electrical and magnetic therapy – it soon became the talk of London. He then opened another health temple in which he installed an elaborate piece of equipment which he called The Celestial Bed. Dr

Graham named this establishment The Temple of Hymen. The name may seem confusing at first, as the word hymen usually refers to (a somewhat evanescent) particular part of the human female anatomy. In Greek mythology, however, Hymen was male. He was the Greek god of the marriage ceremony and if his name was not invoked at an ancient Greek wedding the marriage would prove disastrous. At wedding receptions it was customary for wine-sodden guests to run around shouting his name and praising him.

Dr Graham charged couples £50 a night, a fortune in those days. The silk sheets of the Celestial Bed were purple and the mattress was stuffed with hair from the tails of the finest English stallions. The bed rested on forty pillars of glass and above all the activity was a dome from which issued 'aethereal gases and stimulating aromas'. For the added delight of the bed's occupants the underside of the dome was mirrored and its occupants could also tilt the bed to any pleasing angle. It was surrounded by 1,500 lodestones from which continuously emanated powerful magnetism and throughout the night a pressure pump squirted 'magnetic vapours' which energised the atmosphere surrounding the couple.

In an adjacent room an orchestra played and to encourage the couple, scantily-clad, beautiful young ladies danced erotically around the bed. One of those young ladies was called Emma Lyon. Emma did well for herself. She became Lady Hamilton when she married Sir William Hamilton, the aged British Envoy to Naples. Later she became the mistress of Britain's greatest naval hero, Lord Nelson. Together they formed a bizarre ménage à trois with Sir William offering encouragement from the touchline.

Bellows attached to organ pipes were inserted under the mattress; the volume of musical sounds emitted was in direct proportion to the activity of the couple. The bed was advertised as giving treatment which would 'Insure the removal of the barrenness and invigorate the species of the human being.'

The resourceful James Graham had another scheme up his sleeve; he called it 'Earthbathing.' He set it up in Piccadilly and it was exclusively for women. Ladies, naked but for huge picture hats, would climb into deep vertical pits under his supervision, and then a lad would shovel earth into the pits until the ladies were submerged in earth up to their necks. Dr Graham would then lecture them for forty-five minutes on a variety of medical topics.

Unfortunately for Graham, after a couple of years even the most credulous of London realised that they were being duped, and having amassed sizeable debts (he liked to gamble) he abandoned his London operations and retreated to Edinburgh.

In Edinburgh James Graham delivered frank public lectures on sexual health. These were not at all well received by polite Edinburgh society and he was thrown into Tolbooth jail for two weeks for public indecency.

Towards the end of his days he became religious and took to fiery preaching. Finally his life ended after Earthbathing, himself, every day for many hours, naked, on nine successive days. Thus confirming, if confirmation was needed to an already sceptical world, that Earthbathing was not the great cure-all claimed by Dr Graham.

THROUGHOUT THE AGES THE BRITISH ROYAL FAMILY has provided its loyal subjects with titillating entertainment.. King George III (1738-1820) was pretty conservative when it came to royal flings but his son, George Augustus Frederick (1762-1830), who became Prince Regent, before becoming George IV (1820-1830), was the exact opposite.

George III, known as Farmer George (he kept sheep), distinguished his reign by, in partnership with Lord North, losing the American Colonies and having episodes of madness. He married a German princess, Charlotte of

Mecklenberg-Strelitz. She was ugly with a large mouth, flat nose, and swarthy complexion, and was affectionately known as 'monkey face.' George did his duty by her and the Kingdom, they had eighteen children. Routinely they were in bed by ten o'clock and their court had the reputation of being the dullest in Europe.

The dullest, except when George had one of his outbursts of madness. During episodes he became manic; talked non-stop (once he addressed a tall, stately tree in Windsor Great Park continuously for several hours, believing he was talking to Frederick the Great, the King of Prussia), stayed awake all night, was paranoid and deluded in many ways. A committee of doctors treated him cruelly, but nonetheless in accordance with the accepted medical practices of the time. He needed a strong constitution to survive his doctors' treatments which included repeatedly bleeding him of a basin of blood, purging him, giving him tartar emetic to make him vomit, sedating him with opium, putting him into a straitjacket and strapping him into a specially constructed iron chair, which he rather curiously referred to as 'My Throne.' During manic episodes he developed an embarrassing fancy for an elderly grandmother, Elizabeth Spencer, Countess of Pembroke.

The committee of royal physicians did not appear to make a stab at a proper diagnosis of the cause of George's madness; indeed, a couple of the celebrated physicians of the time appeared to be more concerned with the difficulties they were encountering in collecting their fees. In 1969 research by two distinguished London physicians attributed his madness to an inherited disorder of metabolism called porphyria. But, if only they had known, his servants of the bedchamber were pointing out the diagnosis when they reported that after standing all night the royal wee in the chamber pot had turned a deep purple or black. A diagnostic clue which would not be appreciated for a couple of centuries. More recently, however, some medical historians have thought it more likely that he suffered from bipolar disorder, a manic depressive psychosis.

By 1810 the king's episodic madness had become continuous and was accompanied by rapidly progressing dementia. In the following year George III was declared unfit to rule by Parliament and his son George Augustus Frederick, Prince of Wales, took over as Prince Regent.

A POLE APART FROM HIS FATHER, THE PRINCE REGENT had a long track record of drunken, dissolute behaviour, compulsive sexual conquests, abuse of power, gambling, and spending other people's money like water. He was known as 'Prinny,' and when he was only seventeen he had a passionate adventure with an older lady, an actress, Mary Robinson. The calculating Mrs Robinson knew she had snared a royal goose which would lay golden eggs for her. Prinny had written lovelorn, compromising letters and when the affair ended she charged him £5,000 for their return, Prinny couldn't pay so she turned to his father, George III, who coughed up. She also pocketed an annuity of £500 a year, that had been arranged by Prinny's good friend, the Whig leader, Charles James Fox, who from time to time took over when Prinny tired of an inamorata. Five hundred pounds was a tidy income but, unfortunately for Mary the government frequently neglected to pay her and she sank into penury. She was, however a resourceful lady who took to writing and wrote a best-seller of the day, *Vicenza*.

Despite his all too-numerous encounters with other belles Prinny fell for a devout Roman Catholic lady, the twice-widowed by the age of twenty-five, Maria Fitzherbert. He persuaded her to marry him – convincing her of his seriousness by stabbing himself (not deeply) when she at first declined his offer. The marriage was conducted in secret at midnight in Maria's Mayfair house in 1785 by an Anglican Curate, the Reverend Robert Burt.

Mr Burt was persuaded to conduct the ceremony for a fee of £500; enough to cover his own debt and keep him out of prison. The marriage was void for two reasons; first, he had not obtained the permission of the monarch, his father, in accordance with The Royal Marriages Act 1772, and second, according to The Act of Settlement 1701, as a member of the British royal family, marriage to a Roman Catholic was illegal.

It was just as well that the marriage did not hold up because by the time he reached his late twenties he had amassed enormous debts, £630,000 (£54 million today). His father, George III, refused to ask parliament to pay his debts unless he entered a suitable marriage. 'I'll marry any damn'd German frau!' Prinny declared in desperation.

A first cousin, Princess Caroline of Brunswick was the lucky lady. She had an aversion to washing and a body odour conspicuous even for those days of careless personal hygiene. When Prinny first met her he recoiled in horror and gasped, 'I am unwell. Pray give me a glass of brandy.'

As a footman led him off, Princess Caroline was heard to murmur, 'He's very fat and nothing like as handsome as his portrait.'

At the royal wedding in 1795 the thirty-two year old Prinny was so drunk he had to be held up, and then, while the congregation was kneeling in prayer, he had to be pulled down as he rose, swaying and attempting to make a speech. Princess Caroline confided some days later that he had spent, 'the best part of the bridal night laying under the grate where he had fallen, and where I left him.'

He did, however, manage to clamber into the wedding bed the following morning... as evidenced by the birth of Princess Charlotte of Wales exactly nine months later.

Prince Prinny passed the royal honeymoon in his hunting lodge, Kempshott Park, in Hampshire. He took with him a group of his gambling and drinking cronies and one woman. But, that one woman wasn't his new wife; she was the mistress du jour, Lady Jersey. According to a servant most of the honeymoon was spent with all the men, 'lying around and snoring with their boots on.'

In addition to her noxious odour Caroline had other problems; she was gauche, she enjoyed raunchy stories, she was flirtatious, and she was indiscreet. When she was a teenager her governess was ordered to follow her closely at balls to ensure that she did not have indecent conversations with men. As she aged and gained weight Caroline took to wearing virginal gowns which made her look ridiculous.

In response to Prinny's behaviour, and at the government's suggestion, Princess Caroline took exile in Europe where she was able to tour in style. The government had granted her an annual allowance of £35,000, a large sum for those days, equivalent to about £3 million in today's money. Despite her poor dress sense and malodorous aura (she rarely had her clothes washed and seldom washed herself), she had no shortage of lovers, who no doubt found her title and wealth alluring. One favourite long-term lover was an Italian ex-soldier, a corporal, called Bartolomeo Pergami. The pair became the delight of the cartoonists of London's broadsheets. The embarrassed Prinny attempted to get Parliament to pass an act which would grant him a divorce but when it was pointed out to him that his own infidelities would inevitably be publicised he abandoned the pursuit.

In 1820 Prince Prinny ascended the throne on the death of his father, King George III, and became His Majesty King George IV. That year he again attempted to end his marriage with Caroline and persuaded the House of Lords to pass an act to grant him divorce, but the House of Commons would have none of it. Princess Caroline was immensely popular with the British people and George was hated. Prinny was fifty-seven years old, obese, addicted to laudanum (tincture of opium), and determined to have an extravagant coronation. At vast public expense he had an exact copy of Napoleon's coronation robes made in Paris; it was so heavy it took eight pages to hold the train.

THE CORONATION WAS ARRANGED FOR THE FOLLOWING YEAR, on 19 July 1821. A few days before that date Princess Caroline returned from her European jaunts to take her rightful place as the Queen of England. When she landed at Dover she was greeted by enthusiastic crowds. Despite her coarse nature the British public loved her, equally as much as they loathed her husband.

Prinny's hatred of Caroline was always at the forefront of his mind, so much so that when Napoleon died a couple of months before the coronation and an aide announced, 'Your Majesty, your greatest enemy is dead,'

He replied, with a chuckle, 'Is she, by Jove!'

Naturally he saw to it that Princess Caroline did not receive an invitation to his coronation, nevertheless, she turned up in good time at Westminster Abbey. She was appropriately dressed in a rich red velvet gown wearing a gold crown she had borrowed for the day. At the main door of the Abbey she was refused admission, and when she tried other entrances she was turned away, at one she was refused because she could not produce an entrance ticket.

Within days of the coronation Princess Caroline unexpectedly fell ill. Several times she said that she had been poisoned and in less than three weeks she died of what was called vaguely, 'a gastric disorder.'

After Crown Prince Prinny became His Majesty King George IV, he spent most of his ten-year reign at Windsor Castle. He continued his gluttony, developed gout and grew increasingly obese, so obese that he was deeply embarrassed by it; when he went riding in his coach in Windsor Great Park he would have his footmen clear the public from all the roads ahead.

In 1828 he became short of breath on the slightest physical exertion; he had to be propped up in bed to sleep, and his legs became enormously swollen with oedema fluid – all evidence of heart failure. At a quarter past three in the morning of 26 June 1830 he was holding the hand of his physician when suddenly he gave a start and exclaimed, 'My dear boy! This is death!' and died.

A post-mortem examination showed that the cause of his heart failure was severe aortic stenosis, the aortic valve at the outlet of his heart was calcified and its aperture was grossly narrowed. The cause of him suddenly dying was, however, the rupture of a dilated blood vessel in his stomach, which at autopsy was found to be totally filled with blood.

On balance the death of George IV was celebrated rather than mourned. The Duke of Wellington said that George was, 'The worst man he ever fell in with his whole life, the most selfish, the most ill-natured, the most entirely without redeeming quality.'

And The Times went so far as to write of him that that he, 'would always prefer a girl and a bottle to politics and a sermon.'

Court gossip maintained that during his life every time he bedded a woman he cut off a lock of her hair and sealed it in an envelope with her name on it. It was said that at the time of his death seven thousand such envelopes existed, but none have been found.

A skipping rhyme dating from Prince Prinny's Regency, is chanted by children in England to this day:

> Georgie Porgie, pudding and pie,
> Kissed the girls and made them cry.
> When the boys came out to play,
> Georgie Porgie ran away.

George IV was succeeded by his younger brother William, Duke of Clarence, who was by then sixty years old. He became King William IV and had already sired ten illegitimate children with an actress, Dorothea Jordan, who had four children of her own from previous liaisons. King William IV had no legitimate heir to the throne when he died, so it went to his niece, Victoria. Each of his ten illegitimate children, nevertheless, did well; one was an ancestor of a certain David Cameron, who nearly two hundred years later became the British Prime Minister

3. VICTORIAN SEX – TARTS AND WIVES

TODAY WE ARE BLESSED WITH A VARIETY OF ROLE MODELS FOR OUR YOUTH. The majority are admirable, but there are those who send the wrong message. For example, professional footballers who, with their obscenely high salaries, are less than well behaved on and off the pitch. Role models for adolescent girls are anorexic, skeletal, eccentrically dressed, sullen, pouting, young women who stagger with glazed eyes, ballooned lips, and knock-knees along catwalks. Tattooed, hairy singers of either, or indeterminate sex inspire many of today's youth as they binge their booze and pop their Happiness Pills.

Role models in Victorian times were different; missionaries converting the heathen, second sons forging the Empire with their blood, sympathetic ladies nursing the wounded, and industrial barons employing hundreds; earning millions and endowing hospitals, orphanages, or foundations for fallen women.

Victorian women were bombarded by advice from all sides. The church, lady-friends, moralising pamphlets, magazines, and books especially written for the gentle sex, all conspired to help those delicate, naive souls to fend off their sex-crazed husbands. One scarcely credible piece of advice given to the new Victorian bride was that on her wedding night she should wait for her husband in silence in a darkened room. He would then have to grope his way to the marriage bed, and hopefully, he would stumble and injure himself enough to abandon further proceedings; at least for that night.

Headaches were described as a married woman's best friend but other strategies like starting an argument or nagging him about some trivial household matter just before bedtime would be used to diminish his enthusiasm. Another recommended tactic was to casually mention in the heat of the moment, some ardour-dampening point, like: 'Did you know Darling that our butcher is selling excellent pork pies?'

Or, when hubby had reached an ecstasy of tumescence: 'Looks like rain tomorrow, Dahling!'

The ambition of the middle class Victorian wife, after a decade of wedded life, was to have a stable marriage and four or five children – conceived with a minimum number of procreative acts. She could anticipate that by this stage her husband would enjoy such a comfortable home and agreeable social life that any thoughts of straying would be banished. Even more she would hope that after ten years of frustration he would give up the struggle to have any sort of sex life with her. The watchwords of the Victorian era were: 'Women be Pure! Men be Restrained!'

FRUSTRATED HUSBANDS FELL EASY PREY to the temptations of readily available, inexpensive, gratification with professional or amateur tarts. These encounters often resulted in men picking up a dose of one or other, or both, of the common sexually transmitted diseases, syphilis, and gonorrhoea – and passing them on to their wives, even though sexual contact might be infrequent.

Mrs Beeton, of cookery book fame, was one of those unfortunate wives. She died young, at twenty-eight, and like hundreds of Victorian wives was said to have been infected with syphilis by her husband.

In 1856 each of three of London's many large hospitals recorded dealing with thirty thousand cases of syphilis. The clap (gonorrhoea) was equally common and because it caused a copious penile discharge of pus, the gleet, the diagnosis was easy in men. Gonorrhoea in women could remain symptom-free and undetected, but was nonetheless, highly contagious. It has been estimated that in Victorian times about a fifth of the population was infected with syphilis. The treatment available at that time had little effect on the natural history of those diseases. Not until penicillin arrived nearly a century later was there an effective treatment for either syphilis or gonorrhoea.

Queen Victoria and her consort, Prince Albert, were sexual athletes, always eager but strictly monogamous. The young Victoria seems to have slipped off the pedestal as far as sex is concerned but in other respects she and her husband displayed much of the stuffiness which characterised the period. Disastrously the marriage was cut short when Prince Albert died young. Victoria was only forty-one and from then on dressed in black bombazine. Victoria did not appear in public for three years after Prince Albert's death, and mourned for the remaining forty years of her life. Seeking consolation, she added whisky to her claret at dinner and developed a close friendship with a Scottish gillie, a gamekeeper, John Brown. When he died, Abdul Karim, an Indian Muslim, took over – he taught her Urdu, as well.

The Victorian middle classes were extreme prudes. One example of their prudery was to cover piano legs with trousers lest they provoke fits of lust in men. A second example was that books written by male and female authors should rest on separate library shelves. Mention of an innocent anatomical part like the ankle, or worse the thigh, could send a genteel lady into a swoon. She would then have to be revived with a brain-exploding sniff of smelling salts. All middle-class Victorian ladies carried small green or brown glass bottles of those salts (perfumed ammonium carbonate crystals) in their purses for emergency use.

How come in a decade, the roisterous, hedonistic Regency Georgian days gave way to the restrained Victorian attitudes? The answer can be summed up in two words – 'coal' and 'inventiveness.'

The British Isles were blessed with plentiful supplies of coal and the British people were blessed by having many individuals with inquisitive and inventive minds. The combination of newly developed machines, the fuel to drive them, and the finances of a rich empire led to the British Industrial Revolution. It began in the late 18th century and lasted until the beginning of the 20th century. The Industrial Revolution led to the dominance of the middle class. It was the middle class which determined the sexual reluctance of the so-called weaker sex, and encouraged it to contain the evil lusts of their men.

The country continued, as always, to look up to the aristocracy which consisted of a few hundred families, the Landed Gentry. By divine right the aristocracy governed, established the rules of society, put people in their place and managed the political scene.

WITH THE INDUSTRIAL REVOLUTION, workers in their hundreds of thousands were attracted from the countryside to the towns and cities. These workers formed the lower classes and were supervised by middle class managers. Factories belching smoke needed middle class engineers to manage the cotton spinning and power loom plants. The newly laid railway networks needed middle class administrators. The country became staggeringly rich and naturally such increased wealth expanded the middle class banking industry.

The very face of Victorian England was changed by its ability to manufacture cheap sheet glass, inexpensive paper of good quality, and coal-gas. Gas lights illuminating homes, factories, and streets enabled night to be turned into day and working hours no longer depended on daylight. Industrial chemicals appeared, bleaches for linen mills and sulphuric acid, the most commonly used chemical in many industries, could be made easily and cheaply. The invention of Portland cement revolutionised the building industry.

The increased wealth was paralleled by a population explosion. Between 1801 and 1901 the population of England and Wales doubled to thirty million. More doctors, lawyers, teachers, local government officers, and civil servants swelled the middle class. The middle class became the governing class. The self-made man became a role model. The working class knew its place, so did the aristocracy – the upper class – especially if it landed on hard times and had to go cap-in-hand to the middle class. Industrial barons became barons of the realm when they poured money into the coffers of the political party of the day, but it would take generations for them to lose the cachet of 'trade' in the haughty eyes of the gentry.

While middle class husbands kept their noses to the grindstone their wives and daughters were left to their own devices and developed their own precious society. Not to have a servant, not to have even a 'daily' would be shameful. Aside from producing the next generation, middle class ladies were expected to fritter away their lives, reading books of etiquette and cultivating lady-like manners, they were expected not to deviate one iota from the morals of the Victorian era.

The period was one of self-contradiction; while prostitution and child labour flourished in the working class, and was promoted by the middle class, the middle class embraced sexual restraint, culture and dignity, a strict code of manners, the Anglican Church, and patriotism.

The aristocrats were not concerned with the morals of the nation, as always aristocratic husbands had mistresses and their wives had lovers. The aristocracy continued to rule by divine right. Lord Palmerston, twice Victoria's prime minister, upset Her Majesty by fathering six illegitimate children by different women. He was popularly known as Lord Cupid. At the age of seventy-eight he successfully, and with pride, defended a charge of adultery in which he was the accused and damages amounting to £20,000 were sought.

The year 1840 was eventful. The young Queen Victoria married Prince Albert of Saxe-Coburg-Gotha; the Penny Black stamp was issued to inaugurate the national postal service, and in the United States, William Henry Harrison was elected President. He gave his first (and only) presidential speech on a wet and blustery day, neglected to wear a coat, caught pneumonia, and died within the month. William Goodyear, also in the United States, vulcanised rubber and paved the way for the eventual development of what young American men call 'rubbers' and the British, with a touch of Anglo-Saxon mockery, 'French Letters.'

Also in 1840, William Ewart Gladstone took to the streets of London and set about rescuing fallen women, a task he continued for the next forty years. His activities in the foggy, murky, gas-lit London streets led to suspicions that he might be Jack-the-Ripper, the murderer of Whitechapel prostitutes. Gladstone was prime minister four times during Victoria's reign; she didn't care much for him, she complained, 'He always addresses me as if I were a public meeting.'

TWO YEARS LATER, IN 1842, a young man at Trinity College, Oxford was sent down for neglecting his studies in favour of going to the races. He was Richard Francis Burton, destined to be one of the great Victorian adventurers, one of the greatest travellers in world history and one of the earliest sex tourists. He shocked the Victorian world by his open, inquisitive, and frankly expressed attitude to sex.

He served in the army in India but never rose above the junior rank of captain because he irritated the military authorities with his disrespectful attitude. He was a great writer, linguist, Arabist, explorer, and outraged fellow Victorians by writing copiously about erotica.

Like most European men he found oriental women fascinating. One discovery, recorded in his travel journal, was that if you gave a young oriental lady seven large cloves to chew on the seventeenth day of her menstrual month she would become passionate and insatiable until the end of that month. He gave neither explanation of this fantastic claim nor why starting on the seventeenth was so important.

Burton described the Kabbazah, a technique used by Arab women, whereby during sex the woman would contract her pelvic muscles and give the male member a squeeze. This same technique is widely known today in the Far East as The Singapore Grip; the enjoyment of which can be augmented by a couple of Singapore Slings – a powerful cocktail invented in the Long Bar of the Raffles Hotel, Singapore. It contains gin, cherry brandy, Cointreau, Benedictine, Angostura Bitters, and fruit juices.

Richard Burton had a burning ambition to undertake the Pilgrimage (the Hajj) to Mecca. His Arabic was fluent but he had a problem which could lead to him being unmasked, he possessed a foreskin; that would have to go... so he had himself circumcised. Circumcision was an essential but painful precaution. Should his identity be questioned and his prepuce spotted, he would instantly be revealed as an infidel who had defiled the Holy City, and for sure that would lead to execution.

On one occasion, after he had entered Mecca, he nearly ruined his disguise by standing to urinate. The Prophet

Mohammed had decreed that to prevent soiling their robes Muslim men should squat while passing urine. Burton was observed standing and urinating by a young boy, who was deeply shocked. According to Burton he managed to persuade the boy that he came from India where standing was the custom. Nonetheless, a malicious rumour was spread that to protect his disguise he had killed the boy. This he hotly denied, but the story followed him. Many years later at a formal dinner a fellow guest, a doctor, asked him, 'How do you feel when you kill a man?'

Burton replied roguishly, 'Quite jolly doctor, what about you?'

Burton had an abiding interest in all matters sexual. Some stories stretched credibility, for instance, it was said that wherever he travelled he measured the length of male sex organs and in Karachi he studied the shape of women's breasts. He translated classic eastern works of erotic writings, The Arabian Nights, The Kama Sutra, and The Perfumed Garden. The latter, written by Shaykh Nefwazi, was encyclopaedic and encompassed all aspects of human (and animal) sexual behaviour. To assist men experiencing difficulties the sheikh offered several pieces of advice:

'Men lacking vigour in coition may likewise melt down the fat from the hump of a camel and rub his member with it just before the act; it will then perform wonders and the woman will praise it for its work.'

Shaykh Nefwazi also recommended the aphrodisiac properties of a variety of easily obtained substances, cardamom, ginger, pepper, and oil of lilac. These could be made into to a paste and rubbed in. Less readily to hand, a semi-precious stone, a piece of a blue copper ore, chrysocolla (copper silicate), the size of a mustard seed could be swallowed and was guaranteed to have a miraculous effect. He also wrote: 'The virile member rubbed with ass's milk will become uncommonly strong and vigorous.'

Victorian society was offended by Burton's writings and he in turn was offended by the hypocrisy of Victorian prudery. He adopted an existing (but fictitious) character, Mrs Grundy, a figure of excessive purity and respectability. He used her to mock Victorian society. She was described as the figurehead of The Society for the Suppression of Vice, a puritanical organisation which railed against his writings. But in truth he had no need of Mrs Grundy, the underground world of Victorian pornography was alive, flourishing, and relished Burton's contributions.

Richard Burton had a career spanning twenty-five years in the diplomatic service. He died in 1890 of a heart attack in Trieste. Four years previously Queen Victoria had knighted him for his work as an explorer and diplomat. Whether Her Majesty was privy to his literary works is not known.

Another publication which offended Victorian sensibilities was, The Fruits of Philosophy, a sixpenny book co-published by Annie Besant. She was the divorcée of an Anglican minister, a militant feminist and a liberal humanist. The book advocated birth control and Annie Besant was accused, on that basis, that the book was, 'likely to deprave or corrupt those whose minds are open to immoral injuries.' She was sentenced to six months in jail.

WITH THE INDUSTRIAL REVOLUTION, WORKING CLASS WOMEN for the first time had employment and their own wages; albeit at least a third less than their male counterparts. Factories and the middle class were the largest employers of women. In 1841, with a total population of sixteen million in England and Wales, one million women were in domestic service. Twenty years later a census showed that the proportions had not changed but recorded that three hundred women were now employed in clerical work. It was to take another hundred years and the Second World War for the domestic servant industry to disappear and for women's sexual emancipation to appear – with the invention of the oral contraceptive pill.

These days the delicate, sensitive ladies of the Victorian era have disappeared and in contemporary life, women are approaching equality with men. Sixty percent of entrants to British medical schools are now female. Discrimination on the basis of sex is illegal in western countries. Women fill combat roles in the military. Women vicars are common in the Anglican Church and the gathering of the influential of the Church of England, the Synod, in July 2014 voted approval for the introduction of women bishops.

COULD WOMEN EVER HOLD OFFICE IN THE ROMAN CATHOLIC CHURCH? There is a story (discounted by many religious scholars) that an English woman called Joan – or maybe it was Agnes – went to Rome in the 9th century disguised as a man. She became a priest and was elected Pope by virtue of her learning and sanctity. She was known as Pope John VIII or Pope John Angelicus. The story goes that she became pregnant and the game was up when she went into labour while she was heading a papal procession. She delivered in the street, died, and was buried on the very spot where she had delivered the infant, a boy. A variation of that story is that after delivery she was tied by the ankles to the tail of a horse and dragged through the streets until she died. Yet another variation was that the crowd of shocked onlookers stoned her and the infant to death.

Legend begets legend. It was said that the Church of Rome was so afraid that another woman might be elected Pope that thereafter, when the College of Cardinals had made their final selection, the Pope-elect was required to sit, with naked nether regions, on a chair with a hole in the seat. Then an appointed Cardinal would bend low, avert his gaze and carry out a manual examination – if all was in order he would cry, 'Testiculos habit et bene pendents!' –

He has testicles and they hang well A ludicrous story, and just as unlikely as the story of Pope Joan, but it provided amusement for tittering Protestants.

The Victorian era ended when the eighty-one year old queen died in 1901. She was succeeded by her eldest son who became King Edward the Seventh. Edward had to wait sixty long years to succeed his mother. On more than one occasion he was heard to complain that although everybody prayed to the Everlasting Father he was the only one who had an Everlasting Mother. During his long wait there were parallels between him and King George IV when he was the Prince Regent (Prince Prinny).

Smitten by an aggressive puberty and having a royal title, there could be no holding Edward back from the ladies – or the ladies from Edward. He loved Paris and its houses of pleasure. In one he had his own special room with his royal coat of arms decorating the wall behind the head of the bed. In the centre of that room was a large copper bath which he would have filled with champagne and cavort in it with ladies of the house; it was said that the bubbles tickled the parts and enhanced the pleasures of lovemaking.

Fortunately when he ascended the throne he did not sink into the laudanum-fuelled oblivion of George IV. His frolicking ceased and for the nine years of his reign he turned into a competent and respected monarch. He was much loved, and after he died on the last day of his lying-in-state the queue of grieving subjects was twelve deep and extended for seven miles.

For sure the swooning-prone Victorian ladies would experience near-fatal attacks if they could see their robust sisters of today. The 'weaker sex' now plays soccer in women's leagues and will no doubt in a few years rank alongside men's premier teams… they even play international rugby football… the smelling salts, please.

4. ANNIE ZUNZ CALLED ME BACK

OVER FIFTY YEARS AGO, AT THE AGE OF TWENTY-FOUR, still wet behind the ears and within days of passing my qualifying exams the urge to get to work, doctoring and earning, was overwhelming. Luckily I spotted a card advertising a two week locum tenens post on the jobs' board in the foyer of my London medical school.

I phoned the number on the card and was told the job was mine if I fronted up early the coming Monday morning. Hindsight makes me realise that the hospital was desperate but equally I couldn't wait to swing into action with my recently-examined brain still stuffed to overflowing with medical knowledge and a fancy stethoscope, the latest model, at the ready.

The locum post was for two weeks at the Metropolitan Hospital in Kingsland Road, Hackney. I knew the area, my Uncle Willie lived in nearby Dalston Junction and I had visited him many times. 'Ackney is in London's East End, then it was poor and scruffy, but cockney from its loaf of bread to its plates of meat (cockney rhyming slang, loaf of bread = head, plates of meat = feet). Hackney's row upon row of two-up-two-down, terraced houses were mean with

51

sooty yellow-ochre walls, but its inhabitants as lively and as warm-hearted as the best.

Monday was a sunny, spring morning. I made my way along the busy Kingsland Road which, apart from trolley buses gliding along with a faint whirring noise, looked, for all the world, as it did when Charles Dickens was penning his immortal lines about London's underworld.

The Metropolitan Hospital was opened in 1836 and founded for the treatment of patients whose only recommendations were poverty, destitution and disease. It had a difficult start, for five years it had only five beds and at first this part of London's East End didn't attract rich benefactors.

For a moment I stood on the pavement gazing up at the hospital's austere, grime-encrusted, red-brick facade and paused, wondering what I'd let myself in for. Too late to turn back, I entered, passing through highly polished shining glass swing doors, which contrasted with the otherwise weary appearance of the place.

AS I WALKED THROUGH THE ENTRANCE HALL, a voice behind yelled, 'Oi! Where d'yew think yer goin'?' I turned to see a head wearing a black shiny-peaked cap poking through the porter's window. Superiorly, I announced, 'I'm joining the medical staff.'

Without a word the porter pointed a heavily tobacco-stained index finger at a door marked 'Hospital Secretary'. I knocked, entered, and again thought I was having a Dickensian hallucination… Ebenezer Scrooge was sitting at a littered roll-top desk puffing away at a curved meerschaum pipe and scratching away at a huge ledger. He paused, raised his white-domed bald head fringed with sparse grey hair and gazed at me through gold-rimmed granny spectacles. Removing the pipe and spilling ash on the waistcoat of his black, shiny, threadbare suit he barked, 'Yes?'

'I'm the locum house surgeon.' I responded.

Irritably he brushed hot ash off his soup-stained waistcoat. 'So?'

He looked bewildered as he ran a finger around the inside of a tight, starched, winged collar attached to a once-white shirt. A faded grey cravat held in place with a pearl pin and two-inch stiff cuffs rimmed with black completed the picture. Then light dawned: 'Ah, yes,' he muttered, and scrabbling through the clutter on his desk produced a form with my name on it. With a long bony index finger, sporting a nail edged in jet black, he pointed to a row of dots at the bottom of the page and commanded, 'Sign here.'

Anxious to please, without even a glance at its contents, I did. He also signed, blotted the form and wearily handed it to me saying, 'Here, take this to the porter in the front hall, he'll tell you what to do.'

He reinserted the yellowed stem of the meerschaum between yellowed teeth, returned to the ledger, and dismissed me with a wave of his left hand.

'Mister Larksworthy?' said the porter looking at the form.

'Larkworthy,' I said, 'there is no 's' in my name.'

He handed me a white coat he had taken from a cupboard.

'Here that'll fit yer, that's a funny name you got, though, innit? Come with me Mister Larksworthy – are yer worthy of a lark? Ha! Ha! Come along.'

We ascended a broad flight of stairs, the walls on each side covered by marble plaques recording the charity of long-dead benefactors of the hospital; some had given as much as a hundred pounds, a tidy sum at the beginning of the nineteenth century. Other plaques recorded the gifts of extraordinary donors; the Shoreditch Dance Committee, the Daily Graphic Child Beauty Competition, and the most remarkable of all... His Majesty, The King of Afghanistan. As we passed through glass swing doors at the entrance to a ward I looked up and saw a large notice in letters of gold on a black background, it read: 'Annie Zunz Ward.'

'Mornin' staff,' the porter cheerily said to a staff nurse and wiping the smile off his face as he turned to me, he commanded, 'Wait 'ere,' and left.

The staff nurse looked me over and walked off. As I stood there, bewildered, I wondered, who was Annie Zunz? And what connection did she have with this shabby Victorian Hospital?

I looked around; it was a Nightingale style ward. At that time hospital wards were huge, open, and of the type favoured by Florence Nightingale, a reminder of her design for the Scutari Hospital in the Crimean War which, as it happened, had ended a century before, almost to the day, when I presented myself at the doors of the Metropolitan Hospital.

The ward was rectangular in shape with a nursing station in the middle. Iron beds lined the sides, regimentally spaced and regimentally made up with hospital corners tucked-in tightly at precisely identical angles and not a wrinkle on the starched coverlets. To a height of five feet the walls were tiled in a depressingly dull dark green, and painted above in an even more depressing dingy cream; the woodwork was dark brown. At the far end I spotted a large plaque, it bore a dedication to Annie Sophia Zunz. It was then I remembered that I had seen similar plaques in several London hospitals and even one in my own teaching hospital. Standing there with no idea what to do and musing on Annie Sophia Zunz I was startled by, 'Well! Who are you?' Almost shouted at me, by a fierce, faintly moustachioed, big-bosomed, vast-bottomed, middle-aged lady in a navy blue uniform, with a large, starched, brilliant-white headdress which billowed on each side, looking like the sails of a yacht in a stiff breeze. She was the ward sister.

'I'm the new house surgeon,' I managed timidly.

'Well there are plenty of bloods to be drawn, a couple of electrocardiographs (ECGs) to do and next door on the medical ward there's a lumbar puncture (LP) waiting – the house physician has called in sick. Here are the syringes and specimen bottles, there is the ECG apparatus, and next door the trolley is laid up for the LP. Don't just stand there gawping, get on with it, you don't have all morning; the senior registrar will be doing his rounds in a couple of hours and obviously you know nothing at all about your patients.'

With that she sailed off with her formidable derrière looking like the square stern of a galleon as it plunged and rode a choppy sea.

For a moment I gazed at the kidney dish full of sterile syringes and needles she had handed me. In those days syringes were all glass with the surfaces of the barrels and plungers frosted. Nowadays professional phlebotomists are employed, daily they go around the wards drawing blood samples with an ease born of practice. As a student I hadn't taken that many samples but on my very first morning doctoring I coped – and then disaster. When I came to rinse the syringes the plungers were firmly stuck in the barrels. After I had expelled the blood samples into the specimen containers I should have immediately separated and later washed the plungers and barrels of the syringes before they were sent for re-sterilization. It would be another thirty years before cheap, plastic, disposable, sterile syringes came on the scene. As it was I had ruined five precious syringes, probably costing as much as my week's salary. I recorded the ECGs with difficulty, there was a lot of electrical interference, and soon yards of expensive single-channel ECG recording paper festooned the floor.

I approached the lumbar puncture, my first, with dread. I had witnessed a handful and been taught the landmarks for inserting the long, slim LP needle into the patient's lumbar spine and into the spinal canal. Fortunately the patient was young, flexible and thin. With surprise and delight I succeeded at my first attempt and was able to measure the pressure and collect samples of gin-clear cerebrospinal fluid.

I returned to Annie Zunz ward where I proffered sister the kidney dish laden with blocked syringes and as I did I confessed to the syringe disaster. To my relief she sniffed and all she said was, 'Harrumph,' as she took the dish from my hand. Again, I watched, with pleasure, as that magnificent stern wobbled away.

THE TALL, THIN AND MONOCLED SENIOR REGISTRAR, with his upper lip and nostrils fixed in a permanent sneer, was on loan from St Bartholomew's Hospital. Sporting a mustard yellow waistcoat and a Paisley red bow tie beneath his white coat, he entered the ward with a blast of air and a clunk as the glass doors swung open and closed behind him.

'Morning Sister!' he cried. 'And how's my favourite Sister?'

'Good morning Mr Bentley-Smith,' she simpered. 'We have a new houseman,' she added, sniffing and pointing at me with her chin, 'Mister Larksworthy.'

'Larkworthy,' I murmured, and I heard a small voice in my head say, 'You can always tell a Barts' man… but you can't tell him much!'

'Larksworthy,' he growled.

'Larkworthy,' I corrected.

He ignored me and drawled, 'Where'd you train?'

'University College Hospital,' I replied with pride.

'One of those clever buggers you think yourself, eh?' I shuffled my feet.

'So we'd best get on with it, this first patient here,' he nodded towards and flashed an insincere smile at an elderly lady lying in bed, rigid with fear under a taut, starched coverlet. 'Came in with a strangulated Richter's hernia,' he looked me straight in the eyes. 'What's a Richter's hernia?'

'Sorry, I don't know, sir.'

'You don't know!' he exclaimed, eyebrows raised in exaggerated astonishment as the monocle dropped from his eye and was left dangling on its ribbon.

'Don't they teach you anything at UCH these days?'

The ward round dragged on, the patients were all new to me and the erudite senior registrar took delight in probing for gaps in my knowledge, much as a dentist searching for cavities, and giving a good jab when he found one.

I WAS ON CALL FOR CASUALTY that night and managed, at last, to stagger to bed at about two in the morning. Exhausted, I was asleep the instant my head hit the pillow but I was awakened in half an hour by a rumpus from the room next door. A rich, slurred Irish baritone rendering some anti-English rebel song was accompanied by the noise of crashing furniture and what sounded like a parrot squawking. This went on for half an hour and then after a particularly loud 'Bejaisus'– silence; but only for a minute… then the peace was shattered by stentorian snoring.

Exhausted but irritated I managed to drop off. It seemed only a minute later my shoulder was being shaken. A night porter, Irish as it happened, breathed a gust of tobacco-laden, stale Guinness stout in my face and said hoarsely, 'Theyse wants youse in Cashality.'

Awaiting me there were four young men, all drunk and all with cuts on their faces and hands. Taken by the drink they had had a set-to and used the weapons nearest to hand, bottles and glasses. It took me two hours to sew their wounds and in the meantime they had sobered from the aggressive to the maudlin stage of inebriation. Tearful, forgiving, and bloody they embraced each other and would have embraced me had I not enough residual energy to dodge their loving arms.

Back to bed, five o'clock in the morning; head hits pillow and instantly (actually it was an hour later) same message, same porter, same breath, which in the meantime had been refreshed by a couple of bottles of the black stout. I staggered to Casualty. This time it was a real emergency, a thirty year old man in intense abdominal pain with belly muscles as rigid as a board. I placed the bell of my stethoscope on his belly wall and listened, not a sound, not a suggestion of gut activity. I hadn't seen a case before but it appeared obvious to me that this chap had a perforated ulcer. I called the duty surgeon – I should have guessed who it would be. Of course it was that Barts' senior registrar, Mr Bentley-Smith, but now no bow tie, no monocle, and no waistcoat; instead he wore a dressing gown over striped pyjamas and an irritated frown.

I assisted Mr Bentley-Smith, marvelled at his dexterity and did little myself except hold retractors, mop the surgical field and clip off bleeding points. Very soon he exclaimed, 'There!' and pointed with the tip of a pair of forceps towards a hole the size of a match head on the surface of the duodenum. He closed the hole, over-sewed it with a piece of tissue and closed the abdomen layer by layer. I dragged myself to bed with sore, leaden feet, praying to St Luke, the patron saint of doctors, that I would not experience gusts of Guinness again that night.

The Metropolitan Hospital was under funded and old, its finances didn't even run to a telephone in each room in the doctors' quarters and that was why a night porter would be sent to waken me when I was called. The outpatient department was in the basement, it was dark and gloomy with white tiles from floor to ceiling; the décor was reminiscent of a Victorian public lavatory. Patients and their families crowded together on long wooden benches in a cathedral-like waiting hall.

EVEN THOUGH I WAS A BRAND NEW JUNIOR DOCTOR I was given my own clinic three times a week. My patients were limited to follow-up cases, but many of those were long-service customers with thick dossiers and included a few old lags with an eye for a bit of sport with a callow new doctor. One such told me he had been spitting blood. He produced the evidence, a grubby blood-stained handkerchief; suddenly he spat into it and displayed for me an impressive gobbet of fresh, bright-red blood. Coughing blood is an alarm call. I listened carefully to his chest, his breath sounds were normal and there were no added sounds.

I called in my superior, who was, of course, that sneering senior registrar – he took one look at my patient, smiled and said, 'Hello Bert, coughing blood again are we?' He turned to me, 'Did you look in his mouth?'

Feeling foolish I had to admit that I hadn't. The Barts' man selected a torch and spatula from the examination tray and handed them to me with an unspoken invitation to look into Bert's mouth. There was a laceration on his soft palate, obviously self-inflicted. Looking condescendingly at me the senior registrar said,

'Bert likes us you know, he likes to come here and two or three times has managed to get himself admitted with this and other sorts of fabrications, it's his hobby you see.'

Bert grinned; I felt sheepish.

That night I was not on call. After a supper of cold congealed chips and under-cooked fish in soggy batter in the gloomy hospital canteen I immediately took myself off to bed. As my head hit the pillow I slept, but in the small hours I was awakened once again by the now familiar rumpus next door; squawking parrot, crashing furniture and slurred anti-English rebel ballads.

At breakfast I mentioned this to a senior house surgeon. 'Oh,' he said. 'That's Doctor O'Shaughnessy, the anaesthetic registrar, likes to drink a bit, usually more than a bit and by the time he gets back from the pub his room is kind of unsteady for him, and yes, he does have a parrot in a cage which joins in the fun.'

'But…' I said, 'he's like that most nights.'

'Oh, I see what you're driving at,' said the SHO, 'but he

manages – I guess he just breathes on his first patient to put him to sleep and then takes a few whiffs of oxygen to clear his head.'

He seemed a well-informed sort so I asked him, 'Tell me, do you know who Annie Zunz was? I've seen her name on plaques in the wards of several London hospitals and there's one here in the Metropolitan'

He smiled, 'Annie Zunz? Yes, I happen to know her story.' He paused and cut a slice of rubbery hard, wrinkled fried egg. 'She was an Irish beauty called Annie Sophia Basset. She moved to London where she met and married a German called Siegfried Rudolf Zunz in 1874. Siegfried was an iron magnate, who had come to London in 1860 and made his fortune. Annie died in 1896 after twenty-two years of childless marriage. The broken-hearted Siegfried followed her to the grave three years later. He left a large fortune, to be divided between more than thirty London hospitals, for the construction and upkeep of wards dedicated to the memory of his wife. He stipulated that each ward should be named after Annie and should display a plaque with a dedication to her memory together with a life-sized photograph of his beloved. I must say that although I have seen many of those plaques, I have never seen a photograph of Annie.'

He certainly was a knowledgeable bloke, that senior house officer, and, coincidentally, I met him again twenty years later. At which time he was a specialist surgeon and I was a specialist physician, we were both serving in the Medical Branch of the Royal Air Force.

I learned a lot in those two weeks at the Metropolitan Hospital. I had worked hard and long hours, maybe between seventy and eighty each week. After completing my stint I collected my cheque, a total sum of twelve pounds; which amounted to six pounds a week after deducting four pounds for board and lodging.

TWO WEEKS AFTER ENTERING THE METROPOLITAN hospital and not having left it, not even for five minutes, I departed its walls. On a bright Sunday morning I packed my belongings and as I quit my room, heard snores resonating from my Irish anaesthetist neighbour, doubtless still under the influence of his personal anaesthesia. As I closed my door I realised I had never met him, no matter; heaving a sigh of relief, I walked out of the Metropolitan Hospital for the last time. As I approached the Kingsland Road entrance the head porter stuck his head through the porter's window and called, 'Doctor Larksworthy, there's an emergency on Annie Zunz, go there straightaway.'

'But I don't work here anymore.'

'I can't find another doctor, you'll have to go!' he snapped as he slammed closed the porter's window.

I could have continued walking but my doctor's conscience kicked in. I ran to Annie Zunz and was greeted by an agitated staff nurse who took me by the elbow and led me to a bed in the middle of the ward, ominously the curtains were drawn.

She parted the curtains; I entered, to be greeted by a horrible sight. The patient, the centre of attraction, was a desperately frightened and agitated, elderly, obese lady. She had undergone major abdominal surgery three days before. The large abdominal incision had given way throughout its length and there before my eyes, were her intestines spilled onto the bed.

'You must call the surgeon – immediately,' I told the staff nurse.

'I have,' she wailed, 'but I can't get hold of him and I can't get hold of his registrar, I can't get anybody.'

I LOOKED AT THE PATIENT, HORROR AND FEAR in her eyes; tears on her soft old cheeks, her hands clenched on the sheets, knuckles white. I looked at the distraught nurses, the staff nurse and two probationers. There I was on my own in London, a newly-qualified, junior house-surgeon in a city with hundreds of proper surgeons – but not one to come to my help. The ball was in my court, there was nobody else. I recalled one of my surgical tutors telling the class, 'Remember you will be the one in charge. If you are called to a house where grandpa is sitting on the loo with his prolapsed piles stuck, and in agony – all the family will look to you, you must take charge, you have to remain calm and you have to do something.'

I looked at the patient, the staff nurse, the probationers – they were all staring anxiously at me. I had to do something, it was much more serious than dealing with grandpa's prolapsed piles, but I had to take charge no matter how incompetent I felt... I must remain calm; I must do something but what? For a brief second I thought how overjoyed I would be if that sarcastic senior registrar would throw open the doors of Annie Zunz and stride into the ward. With an immense effort I controlled myself.

'Right, Staff Nurse, bring me plenty of sterile swabs; sterile drapes, sterile gloves, the strongest suture material you have with a big round needle. Bring me a large syringe, needle, and local anaesthetic but first of all I will give her a shot of intravenous morphine, so open the Dangerous Drugs Cupboard and get me an ampoule – you do have the key, don't you?' Relieved, she nodded, and ran to the cupboard.

The morphine injection, minimal though it was, calmed the old soul quickly and after cleaning the skin with an antiseptic and draping the area I infiltrated the wound edges with local anaesthetic. Carefully and gently I replaced the abdominal contents and then brought the wound edges together, sutured them and applied a sterile dressing. To support the abdominal wall I firmly applied a many-tailed bandage. I turned to the Staff Nurse. 'That should do as a temporary fix, but you must keep trying to get hold of the senior registrar.' With that I turned and left the hospital.

RUPTURED ABDOMEN IS A SERIOUS COMPLICATION following major surgery and the outlook is not good. The proper way to treat a ruptured abdomen and give the best chance of survival is to take the patient to the operating theatre and under general anaesthesia close the abdominal wall with massive, full-thickness sutures. I have sometimes wondered what happened to that poor old lady; no doubt long dead after all this time… but hopefully she had a few good years after my amateur surgery.

And what happened to the Metropolitan Hospital? It closed as a hospital in 1977. At first the building housed the homeless and was called the Metropolitan House Hostel. Subsequently it became accommodation for young French, Spanish, and Italians coming to London to work. A French girl was murdered there in 2006.

5 BRUSHES WITH THE LAW

MY FIRST CAR

REMEMBER YOUR FIRST CAR? Everybody remembers their first car and its registration number. Mine was registered in Cornwall in 1939 and its registration number was FAF 676. It was an Austin Eight, twenty years old (six years younger than me) when I bought it in 1959. I paid £165 for it – equivalent to about £3,000 today. At the time I had completed my first year as a junior doctor and was a senior house officer to the Plymouth hospitals group.

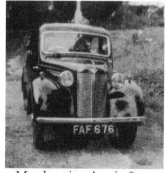

My gleaming Austin 8

That car was my pride and joy. Of course it was black; there was no choice in those austere days. To me it had fine lines; unblemished chromium in profusion, leather upholstery, a varnished wooden dashboard and, most important, it had the magical smell of a car. I kept it highly polished and decorated the radiator with the badges of the British Medical Association and the Automobile Association.

There are precious few of us still around who can remember those Automobile Association patrolmen riding their bright yellow motor cycles and sidecars. They were as smartly uniformed as any Nazi Gestapo Gauleiter, as they cruised the highways. If they encountered a motorist sporting the AA badge they would snap a smart salute with their right hand, which was invested by a large leather gauntlet. The salute was not just to give members a feeling self-importance – it was more important, it could give a warning – if the patrolman did not salute there was a speed trap around the corner.

That Austin 8 was delicate, starting her was an art. There was a knob on the dashboard, labelled 'choke,' which when pulled out would enrich the fuel/air mixture, but too much choke and the engine flooded, the car filled with petrol fumes and there was no alternative but to hang around until the excess petrol in the carburettor had evaporated. My Austin was not powerful but I found that she had a taste for a brand of petrol long since defunct, National Benzole Superior. If her tank was filled with that brand as I drove out of the filling station she would practically rear up on her hind legs. It was one shilling and ten pence a gallon – about two new pence a litre – back then those life-giving liquids, petrol and beer, were remarkably cheap.

Mind you, she wasn't a fast lady; to get her up to sixty miles an hour required priming by starting the run downhill. One of my embarrassing moments with her occurred when I was travelling across Salisbury Plain, trailing a motor coach. Signalling that the road ahead was clear, the friendly driver waved me on. I pulled out and accelerated, but even with the pedal-to-the-metal I could not pass that coach which was doing a steady fifty miles an hour. A bunch of schoolchildren crowded the rear window, they were watching me, urging me on and pulling faces – to my embarrassment, and their delight – when a car appeared, approaching rapidly in the opposite direction, I had to brake and drop back.

She wasn't keen on the cold and like many members of the fair sex took a bit of starting; sometimes I had to resort to a hand job, always remembering, as I cranked the engine, the Chauffeur's Fracture. This happens when you let go of the starting handle at the end of the swing and it instantly springs back giving your wrist a mighty whack.

ONE MORNING I PARKED IN THE BUSTLING CENTRE OF PLYMOUTH, it was Market Day and the car parks were full. With a skill, which surprised me, I managed to insert my Austin into a gap in a line of cars, each parked with two wheels on the pavement. Illegal I knew, but what the heck? There were plenty of cars in front and behind.

When I returned half an hour later, to my horror, I found my car in solitary splendour... guiltily I looked around; the coast was clear, I got in turned on the ignition and was about to pull the starter button when from nowhere PC 149 appeared, looking bright and alert, the silver on his bobby's helmet gleaming and its black strap embracing his chin. The buttons of his uniform were shining and he was wearing a 'Gotcha!' expression on his face. He tapped on the window, I wound it down and he said, 'Young man you are parked illegally.'

I replied, as innocently as I could, 'I'm very sorry, officer, when I parked there were cars in front and there were cars behind and I thought that restrictions were lifted on market days.'

Of course I knew I was in the wrong, and he knew I knew. He did not seem at all impressed when I replied that I was a senior house officer at the local hospital, in response to his enquiry asking what I did for a living. He proceeded to give me a lecture on parking my car properly at all times; on my civic duties in general, on respect for the truth and so on. His lecture lasted a quarter of an hour and while he pontificated I held my tongue. Eventually he let me go having emphasised that he was a generous, kind-hearted bloke and would get no pleasure in hauling me before the magistrates, who would undoubtedly fine me a fiver. I thanked him for being such a kind and considerate member of the human race and reassured him of my newly-found, and deep respect, for the law.

AT MIDNIGHT A WEEK LATER I WAS ON CALL and was summoned to the Casualty Department. The rumpus could be heard a mile away. In a cubicle with a couple of policemen there was a drunk; he was creating havoc and being restrained by the two cops. One of the cops was my old friend, PC 149, who instantly recognised me and greeted me like an old pal. 'Hello doc, how are you? We think this man has injured himself and needs to be admitted, he is causing all sorts of mayhem in the lock-up.'

I was accompanied by a burly male nurse and asked the policemen to leave us and have a cup of tea while I examined the drunk. As soon as the cops left the cubicle the drunk calmed down. He was very drunk but there was no evidence of head or other injury when I examined him. The nurse called the policemen and as soon as they appeared our man started his shenanigans again. Suppressing a smile I told them that he was just drunk and could be taken back to the police cells.

'But,' I added, 'keep a close watch on him, one of you must sit with him all night, you're right he could injure himself.'

With that I bade the policemen good night, smiled warmly at my friend, PC 149, and left.

WAS HE CLINICALLY DRUNK?

ONE NIGHT AS DUTY DOCTOR at a Royal Air Force base in Northern Germany I was called in the small hours to attend to an airman who had been brought in having been involved in a fight in the local village tavern.

In an alcohol-fuelled set-to with another airman he had been slashed three times across the face with a broken glass. The lacerations criss-crossed but although there was considerable bleeding, the cuts were not very deep. There was no indication that an artery had been severed, and there was no evidence of facial nerve damage. He was drunk, bordering on coma, and minimal local anaesthesia was needed during the hour it took to carefully suture his wounds.

When ten days later I removed the stitches, the results of my handiwork were pretty good, I was pleased – and so was he. I advised him to take care in the future and to remember that, although resembling fizzy pale-brown lemonade, many German beers were much stronger that those he was accustomed to drinking in England.

I thought no more of the incident until two months later I was notified that I would be required to appear as a witness at the court martial of the airman who had assaulted my patient.

On the appointed day in number one dress uniform, with buttons shining I appeared in the ad hoc court room on the base – a lecture theatre in the Education Section. I saluted the Judge Advocate; I was sworn in and told to remove my cap and to sit down. Then I was addressed by the prosecutor. He was a Queen's Counsel, a big man with a booming voice. He was wearing a wig and a black gown which he hitched up repeatedly when, every thirty seconds, it slipped off his right shoulder.

'DOCTOR,' he addressed me. 'You treated the victim of the accused?' I agreed that I had done so.

'Please tell the court what diagnosis you made and what treatment you gave.'

'He had three lacerations on his face, fortunately they were superficial and there was no evidence of damage to the facial nerve or arteries. I sutured the wounds under local anaesthesia.'

'Thank you, doctor.'

The QC hitched his gown once more, and asked, 'And what was the mental state of your patient?'

'He was clinically drunk.' I replied.

WHEREUPON THE LEARNED JUDGE LEANED TOWARDS ME and, peering over his gold-rimmed, half-moon spectacles, said in a testy tone, 'DOCTOR, drunk is drunk, there's no such thing as clinically drunk, anybody can tell if a person is drunk, you don't have to be a doctor to make the diagnosis; the whole world can see if a person is drunk, you don't need a medical degree, clinically drunk is nonsense!'

The QC hitched up his gown and said, 'Well?'

'He was drunk.' I said.

A TRAGIC CASE.

I WAS LEAVING A ROYAL AIR FORCE HOSPITAL, at lunchtime, when the receptionist called me back. 'There's an emergency on the paediatric ward, a child has collapsed!'

I ran the hundred and twenty yards to the ward and found that a girl of seven, who had just returned from the Recovery Room after a tonsillectomy, had suffered a cardiac arrest. I checked that the nurses were following the correct resuscitation procedures and quickly hooked the girl to a heart monitor... the tracing was flat. The crash cart was standing by and I gave an injection of adrenaline directly into her heart. In a matter of twenty seconds we were delighted to see a flutter on the trace and then the normal heartbeat resumed. By this time the anaesthetist, who had administered the anaesthetic during her tonsillectomy, had arrived and took over. I departed.

I later heard that the little girl had suffered such severe brain damage during the period her heart was not beating, that she was intellectually and physically crippled, to such an extent that she would need twenty-four hour nursing care for the remainder of her life.

A year later I was told that the parents were taking action against the Ministry of Defence claiming that negligence had led to their daughter's cardiac arrest, I would be called as a witness in the action and representatives of the RAF Legal Branch would come to the hospital the following week to take a statement from me.

Taking that statement took a whole day. The length of the corridor was carefully measured and the time it took for me to run to her bedside from the Hospital Reception was measured – three times I had to do that run. My statement was typed up and I signed it.

SIX MONTHS PASSED AND I WAS told that the case was to be heard in the Family Division of the Royal Courts of Justice in the Strand in London. I was also told that witnesses were to assemble in a certain barrister's chambers the evening before in order to be briefed by the defending council.

There were six of us sitting around a brilliantly polished large mahogany table in the conference room of the chambers. The barrister was dressed in a smart three piece Savile Row black suit with remarkably broad chalk stripes. He was tall, imposing, middle aged, and very fat, with a gold watch chain stretched across his ample, tense abdomen. Conscious of speaking to an audience of inferior mortals and aware that we all had blighted intellects he spoke slowly with pomposity and an affected upper-crust accent. After a couple of hours he came to my evidence, read it through and asked me, 'Why do you think she suffered brain damage?'

'Because her heart had stopped and that resulted in cerebrovascular insufficiency.' I replied.

He looked down his nose and said pompously, 'Just what do you mean? Cerebrovascular insufficiency, what in heaven's name is cere-bro-vas-cu-lar insufficiency?'

I was about to reply when – sitting next to me – the Royal Air Force Civil Consultant Adviser in Cardiology, an eminent Harley Street physician, also irritated by the barrister's pomposity, touched my arm, leaned forward and said.

'What the Wing Commander says is very simple; he is using English words with which we are all familiar.' He paused. '"Cerebro," to do with the brain, "vascular," to do with the blood supply, "insufficiency," not enough.' He looked the pompous, learned counsel in the eye and repeated, 'Not enough blood was getting to the child's brain – there, do you get it now?'

Counsel was deflated. 'Yes,' he muttered as he gathered up his papers, and with a gruff 'See you all tomorrow in Court number three at ten in the morning,' swept out.

WE ASSEMBLED AS INSTRUCTED AND ALL STOOD when the bewigged judge in a red robe entered; he bowed to the court and sat down, we took our seats. The surroundings were intimidating; I was feeling nervous, picturing myself being aggressively questioned by the prosecution, yet another eminent Queen's Council.

I need not have worried. Within seconds of the judge sitting down the prosecuting and defending barristers approached the bench and had a few words. After a couple of minutes the court was adjourned for an hour.

The cardiologist and I crossed the Strand to a cafe and ate doughnuts and drank coffee for half an hour. When we returned we learned that the case had been settled.

I was relieved that I wouldn't be cross-examined but disappointed that I didn't get to witness our pompous QC battling it out with an equally pompous QC for the plaintiffs.

THE ALL-POWERFUL SUBORDINATE
COMMANDER

WHEN I WAS POSTED TO MALAYSIA AS A SENIOR SPECIALIST in internal medicine I had held the rank of Squadron Leader for five years. I had no idea that I was the senior Royal Air Force officer based in Peninsular Malaysia.

One morning, in the middle of a clinic, there was a loud knock on my consulting room door and in marched an RAF flight sergeant policeman who came to attention, saluted and said, 'I have to inform you, sir, that you will be required to hear a formal charge concerning an airman.'

'What me?'

'Yes, sir, you are the senior ranking officer in this Command."

'But I know nothing about RAF law and I have no idea of legal procedure.'

'It's a very simple case, sir; one of the lab technicians has lost his 1250. We'll do it tomorrow.'

'Tomorrow?'

'Yes, tomorrow, sir, best get it over quickly, we'll front up in the morning at eleven sharp.'

'Thank you, flight sergeant.' I replied.

I read up what seemed relevant in the copy of 'The Manual of Law for the Royal Air Force,' the hospital adjutant held in his office; it seemed simple enough. The form 1250 is a serviceman's identity card and its loss is regarded as a serious matter.

I was sitting in my air-conditioned office the next morning when promptly at eleven there was a clattering of boots and a voice shouting, 'Left!Right! Left!Right! Sharp Left!'

There was a loud bang on my door. 'Come in!' I cried, and the door was flung open.

A corporal policeman entered, followed by the 'criminal' and the flight sergeant. They lined up in front of me saluted and the flight sergeant read the charge.

'Junior Technician Evans; charged with loss of Royal Air Force Form of Identity Twelve-Fifty. Hat off! Attenshun!'

I sat there wearing my service dress cap, desperately trying to look serious. I knew Evans; he was a good laboratory technician, a happy-go-lucky Welsh lad. I squirmed in my seat, I had never understood 'squirming in one's seat' but I did then, as I shifted from one buttock to the other trying to keep a severe face.

'Well, Evans?' I demanded. 'How did this happen?'

'Don't know, sir, found I'd lost my ID when I returned from a night out in Penang.'

That appeared to be it, there were no other charges and he had an unblemished record.

'Will you accept my punishment?' I demanded.

'Yes, sir,' he replied without a trace of apprehension.

'Junior Technician Evans, I hereby admonish you for the loss of your Identity Card, form 1250, and I award you one month's extra duties.'

Evans accepted and signed the form.

'Hat on – AT-TEN-shun! Salute! About turn - quick march!' screeched the flight sergeant.

I completed the paperwork, signed it and off it went to the Provost Marshal's office in Singapore.

A week later I took a call in the middle of a busy clinic. It was from headquarters in Changi, Singapore. A very uptight Legal Branch wing commander barked, 'What the bloody hell are you up to Larkworthy?'

'What's the problem?' I asked.

'PROBLEM? PROBLEM!' he shouted. 'You have

awarded two punishments for one offence; extra duties is a punishment and so is an admonishment. And what's more you can't award extra duties to an airman, only to a boy entrant. This whole damn nonsense is quashed.'

With that he slammed down the phone and I felt abashed – just a little.

I went to the laboratory as soon as I could and told Evans what had happened. He was happy that no entry would blot his record and when I added that he had no extra duties because of 'an administrative error' he said nothing but gently smiled from ear to ear.

About a week later I was in the path lab looking down a microscope for evidence of malaria in some blood smears when Evans sidled up to me and said quietly,

'Me and the lads were wondering – when can we have another court martial?

,

6. WHEN I PLAYED CRICKET FOR ENGLAND

IN 1970 I PLAYED CRICKET FOR ENGLAND AGAINST AUSTRALIA. It wasn't in England at Lords or the Oval, or in Australia, in Sydney or Melbourne, it was in Malaysia.

The match was held on the sports ground of the Royal Australian Air Force Base at Butterworth in Province Wellesley on the mainland of Malaysia, opposite the beautiful island of Penang, 'The Pearl of the Orient.'

At the end of 1968 I was posted to Malaysia on loan to the RAAF Hospital as the senior physician; the Australian military having no full-time serving medical or surgical specialists. Although we Poms were outnumbered by ten to one by the Ozzies on the hospital staff we could not ignore a challenge to play a local Test Match when, towards the end of a well-lubricated Dining-In Night, the Australian Hospital Commanding Officer threw down the gauntlet. At that time England had surprisingly beaten Australia in a Test Match and we Brits were given over to a good deal of crowing. We just managed to scrape together a team by including a couple of not-too-willing female,

English, Princess Mary's Royal Air Force Nursing Officers; also on loan service.

On the day the most important man of the match rode a bike around the field. He delivered sustenance to batsmen, fielders, and umpires from the handlebar basket filled with cans of ice-cold Tiger beer. Local rules dictated that each 'event' in the game was accompanied by a swig of beer. 'Events' included boundaries, the fall of a wicket, a nice piece of fielding, or a failed 'Owzat!' There would be a pause while refreshing draughts were taken, then the batsmen would place their cans behind the stumps, the fielders stood their cans at their feet, the umpires put them in a pocket of their white laboratory coats and play resumed.

To begin with we were worried that the sides were desperately and unevenly balanced – but our anxieties came to nothing. The Aussie batsman we most feared, the flight lieutenant hospital adjutant, had played for Queensland, but after he had swallowed a few 'tinnies' of Tiger he became, like all of us, as equal as the citizens in any Marxist regime.

My memory of the end of the match is blurred. I can't recall the result but I remember chaos reigning at the end. The beer delivery man fell off his bike, my medical registrar (who was a big, strong and very tight Australian) picked up his wicket-keeper, who had dropped quite a few simple catches, and holding him horizontally, ran the twenty-two yards between the wickets to throw him at the stumps at the other end, amid cheers and the clanking of a pile of empty beer cans. That done, and a somewhat slurred speech by the Group Captain Commanding Officer congratulating both sides for a game played in a true sense of Anglo-Australian animosity, we retired to a bar on the beach facing Penang. The beauty of the sunset with its usual technicoloured panorama of the cloud-wreathed island of Penang contrasted with bawdy British and Australian ditties which needless to say had themes much in common – lusty lads have the same thoughts no matter which hemisphere.

BUTTERWORTH IS IN PROVINCE WELLESLEY, both British names for places in the Malaysian Peninsula. The town was named after William T. Butterworth who was governor of Singapore and Malacca from 1843 to 1855; the Province was named for Arthur Wellesley, the Duke of Wellington.

In my day, over forty years ago, Butterworth had a population of a hundred thousand; smelted tin, made sweet and sickly biscuits and bottled fierce chilli sauce. It had the smelliest drains in Southeast Asia and smelly markets to compete with the drains. Large piles of fly-ridden fish and prawns dried in the tropical sun and in season the vile smell of the durian fruit was all-pervasive.

The durian is a large spiked tropical fruit with a thick yellow-green skin. It contains a creamy flesh with large seeds. The smell has been likened to that of rotting strawberries in a badly kept public lavatory – but the taste? For those who can get beyond the noxious smell (I wasn't one) the taste is said to be divine. It also has the reputation of being an aphrodisiac and when the large ripe fruits fall from a tree and land with a thump, the locals, each time excited by the sound, say with a twinkle in their eyes, 'When the durians are down! The saris are up!'

I looked after Australian and British forces and their families. It was an exciting and interesting time, made the more interesting by also taking care of Gurkhas and their families. The Gurkha soldiers were stationed in two centres in the Malaysian peninsula; at Minden Barracks on Penang Island and on the mainland at the training depot at Sungei Patani, a town near Ipoh, some fifteen miles north of Butterworth.

Gurkhas are special, they are the most loyal and fearless soldiers Britain has ever had. Friendly, with a raunchy sense of humour, their discipline is impeccable. Even as patients in hospital they show intense discipline; if on ward rounds a sick Gurkha did not jump out of bed and stand to attention, or at least come to attention as he lay in bed – I would know he was really sick.

Many times I had to admit Gurkhas in groups because they not infrequently acquired medical problems in groups. Platoons collectively picked up infections on jungle patrol – the commonest was malaria with scrub typhus and Weil's disease close behind. Fever is non-specific but heralds the onset of each of those infections. It is essential to differentiate rapidly between the illnesses because of their serious nature and because, although treatment for each is rapidly effective, it is quite different.

The history often gave the clue; malaria – had the platoon commander forgotten to take a supply of malaria prophylaxis tablets? Scrub typhus – had the platoon spent the night in the relative comfort of a deserted jungle village? The nasty bug which causes scrub typhus has the exotic name Orientia tsutsugamushi. Its reservoir is in mites which live on rats which colonise the barasti of abandoned huts. The mites jump off the rats and bite and infect the sleeping soldiers. The third, Weil's disease is caused by bacteria (Leptospira icterohaemorrhagiae) harboured by river rats and excreted in their urine. If a soldier crossing a river on a rope bridge dropped his rifle the platoon would enjoy a refreshing hour diving and looking for it. The different diagnoses were quickly indicated by the history and the clinical examination and confirmed by the results of simple, rapid laboratory tests.

AN UNUSUAL PROBLEM OCCURRED ONE MONDAY morning when a Gurkha presented with a paralysed right wrist. He brought a letter from his unit army medical officer which told me that this mysterious paralysis had suddenly appeared in their stores' officer, Warrant Officer Prambahadur Rai, on Sunday morning.

The diagnosis was obvious – he had a Saturday-Night

Palsy. After I examined him I asked, 'Warrant Officer were you drinking on Saturday night?'

'No doctor sahib,' he replied, mortally affronted, 'doctor sahib; I do not drink.'

'You do not need any treatment,' I told him.

'No treatment doctor sahib?'

'Yes, no treatment, this will recover on its own, come and see me again in a week.'

He looked puzzled. 'No treatment doctor sahib?'

'No, no treatment, come back in a week.'

He stood rigidly to attention but couldn't salute because his wrist was paralysed.

'Thank you doctor sahib,' he said, with doubt in his voice.

When he appeared a week later he snapped a salute, the paralysis had recovered. He stood before me holding his left hand behind his back and asked, 'Doctor sahib; how you know I drink? I had taken very big lot of rum.'

'Well, Warrant Officer, I know about these things and I know that what you had sometimes happens with plenty, plenty rum (the Gurkhas' favourite tipple). And remember this Warrant Officer Prambahadur Rai, it is useless not to tell the truth to a doctor sahib.'

Warrant Officer Prambahadur Rai then produced a kukri, the Gurkhas' traditional weapon, a large curved knife, almost the size of a small sword, from behind his back and handed it to me saying, 'This is for you, doctor sahib, I am very sorry, I lied.'

SATURDAY NIGHT PALSY OCCURS when the victim, bordering on alcoholic coma, falls asleep with his arm over the back of a chair. For many hours, throughout the night, there is unremitting pressure on the nerve which controls the muscles which extend the hand at the wrist. Anatomically speaking the nerve runs down inside of the upper arm and lies between the humerus bone and the hard chair back. When the patient wakens he finds to his hung-over horror that his wrist is paralysed. Invariably recovery is spontaneous, it's just like a nerve of sensation which has 'gone to sleep' returning to life in a matter of minutes after the pressure is released, but a Saturday night palsy takes a few days.

I still have that kukri. The sheath is made of ox hide, the handle of ox horn and two additional small blades are incorporated, one to sharpen the wicked curved blade and the other a small knife. Tradition dictates that once drawn a kukri cannot be re-sheathed unless blood is drawn. That is when the small knife proves useful… to nick a finger to obtain a bead of blood.

Gurkhas enjoy life to the full; they thrive on soldiering, partying, and a particular religious festival, the Dashera, the culmination of which involves the beheading of a buffalo. I attended a Dashera Fest held at the parade ground in the training depot at Sungei Patani.

On a brilliant sunny October morning I was seated with other guests on a dais with the officers and their wives. The Depot Commanding Officer, a full colonel, sat in the middle of the front row with his lady wife on his right and the Gurkha Officer Commanding, a Queen's Commissioned Gurkha Major, on his left. The parade ground was surrounded by soldiers, their wives and a large number of highly excited children.

The climax of the ceremony, and its main objective, was to execute a buffalo by chopping off its head with one clean slice. More than one chop or an incomplete operation with even the most slender piece of tissue linking head and neck would be counted a failure, and doom and gloom would follow… for a year.

The instrument used was what looked like an overgrown kukri and was called a kukruji. A very muscular Gurkha dressed in a white loincloth was standing at attention and holding vertically the sharp sword with its blade glinting in the sun. To test the sharpness of its cutting edge a large papaya on four wooden stilts was placed a few yards in front of the dais, the kukruji was raised and lowered gently until the sharp edge touched the fruit. Then with no pressure and simply by its own weight and razor sharpness the blade descended through the large fruit and, to enthusiastic clapping, the cleanly cut two halves fell apart.

He then executed half a dozen chickens, whipping off their heads at lightning speed and throwing the headless bodies, which ran amok spurting blood, into groups of excited children who screamed with delight. When the commotion subsided he practised on larger sacrificial objects, a couple of sheep and three goats. All were despatched with consummate ease.

Finally the reluctant buffalo was dragged onto the parade ground by six uniformed soldiers. Using ropes and considerable effort the head was tied to a stake the width of a telegraph pole which had been, prior to the ceremony, sunk into the middle of the arena. Then with all six soldiers standing to the beast's rear and pulling on its hind quarters its neck was stretched – the buffalo's head, with bulging, rolling eyes, was held immovably attached to the stake… the neck was taut – everybody held their breath.

The sword flashed; the neck was completely severed, we all cheered, and triumphantly the soldiers, pulling on the ropes attached to the buffalo's headless body, dragged the carcass around the parade ground – blood spouting with diminishing force as the heart, progressively deprived of blood, failed and stopped.

The Gurkha, who had performed so well, approached the dais and stood to attention. The colonel descended, shook him by the hand and tied a ceremonial white turban around his head. Relieved, we repaired to the Officers' Mess where trays of glasses filled with whisky awaited our pleasure. After two or three we enjoyed a curry buffet prepared Gurkha style.

The tough Gurkhas always ate the liveliest of curries; even what appeared to be a simple boiled potato could burn a hole in your palate. Chicken were prepared without fuss. Most of the feathers would be taken off and then the cook with his cleaver; starting just aft of the beak, would chop, chop, chop, finishing a couple of centimetres above the claws. I never found the courage to enquire about the viscera.

MY TOUR IN MALAYSIA CAME TO AN END IN 1971. I would have willingly spent longer with those marvellous soldiers and their families. It so happened that, a couple of weeks before I was due to leave, the Training Depot at Sungei Patani was closing and being transferred to Hong Kong. I attended The Beating of the Retreat to mark the end of that era in the history of the Gurkha Regiment. Two whimsical memories of that ceremony remain with me.

The first, as the kilted Gurkha pipe band in full Scottish military uniform played and the troops marched and counter-marched in impeccable order, the express steam train, from Singapore to Bangkok via Butterworth, passed by in the distance and, deliberately or not, the driver gave two loud long wailing hoots. The other memory; I was sitting immediately behind the colonel's lady when a large bee got itself entangled in her chignon, she was unaware of its struggles and I was on the point of leaning forward to alert her when it freed itself and flew away – symbolic I thought – time for all of us to go.

7. MANY A SLIP

SOON AFTER I QUALIFIED, AND WITHIN DAYS OF STARTING MY FIRST PROPER JOB, as a house surgeon in a big, busy general hospital, I experienced for the first time the death of a patient under my care. It was my first patient death as a doctor and, although I had encountered death many times in my student years, I was upset.

I had looked after Charlie Brown, a relatively young man of fifty-five, for about ten days. He had suddenly and unexpectedly died three days after surgery and, as it happened, immediately before afternoon visiting hours. I phoned my boss, the consultant surgeon, to inform him and was perturbed when he said we needed a post-mortem examination to find out exactly what had gone wrong. 'Speak to the family, Larkworthy,' he said, 'explain why we need the examination; I'm sure you'll get their permission with no bother.'

A sympathetic staff nurse intercepted Mrs Charlie Brown and her son as they were about to enter the ward and took them to Sister's office. I was called and sat down with them, the ward maid brought tea and biscuits. I explained that her husband had undergone long and difficult but apparently successful surgery but that post-operatively, something had suddenly and disastrously gone wrong.

Their faces dropped, the new widow wept; the shocked son looked at me and said, 'So what's to be done doctor?'

'We need to do a post mortem examination so that we can find out exactly what had occurred and to determine if there was an unforeseen complication, so that in future we may be able to avoid what happened to Mr Brown happening in others,' I replied, thinking that I had neatly summarised the problem.

'B-But,' stammered the son. 'Our name is Jones.'

I was talking to the family of the patient in the bed adjacent to the one who had died.

A FEW YEARS LATER I FOUND MYSELF in a Yorkshire mining town near Barnsley. I was doing a locum for two weeks for the local single-handed general practitioner. He was so exhausted he was simply taking two weeks holiday at home with his feet up and indulging in the luxury of consecutive nights of undisturbed sleep.

I quickly came to understand how he could be so exhausted. This was about a dozen years after Aneurin Bevan had launched his National Health Service, promising free spectacles, free false teeth, free round-the-clock access to doctors and nothing to pay at the point of service – there is nothing the Yorkshire folk find more attractive than the concept of, 'summat for nowt' and they were running their doctor ragged.

My morning surgeries, especially on Mondays, had no less than sixty patients of both sexes, many of them healthy but just hung-over and demanding sick notes. At first I felt it my duty to point out that they were not suffering an illness which should keep them off work, but this took time and some responded with Yorkshire belligerence to this young, know-it-all, toffee-nosed doctor from the South. In the end I had to quash my qualms, sign the sick note, and get on with the next patient. Almost invariably towards the conclusion of an exhausting surgery dealing mostly with trivia there would be two or three really sick patients with serious problems, like pneumonia or heart failure.

Night calls were a burden. I was on call every night and every night I was called out at least twice. Some so-called emergencies could be handled on the phone. Often I was called with trivial complaints, one memorable phone call was at three in the morning, I had already been called twice from my bed, and a loud, broad Yorkshire female voice told me, 'Me clacker's on fire an' it's itching laik buggery.'

Although an ignorant southerner it took only a few seconds and a couple of questions to understand that she had a dreadful itch affecting her private parts.

'So what's to do?' She demanded aggressively.

In my exhausted state I could only think of one response: 'Scratch it!'

When I later told that story to a Scottish gynaecologist colleague she said, 'Och, you shouda told her to slap yoghurt on it, vairy soothing, an aw.'

Again the smart-alec response – 'Any particular flavour?'

LATE ONE AFTERNOON, TACKLING THE LAST OF THE MORNING'S house calls, I was at a run-down council house seeing a run-down elderly lady with a pain in her neck. She was sitting at one end of a dining table, at the other end sat an old chap rolling his day's supply of cigarettes and enveloped in a cloud of the foul smoke of cheap, roll-up tobacco. The room was hot; the fire was heaped with burning coals, it was a mining town, coal was free.

The old fellow was toothless and wore an off-white shirt with a stud at the neck, grey frayed braces and a greasy flat cap, which I guessed adorned his head night and day. As usual the television in the corner was blaring and nobody was watching it. When I first entered the room with a cheery, 'Hello, good afternoon,' he had ignored me. He continued to ignore me as I examined and then discussed treatment with the patient. I wrote a prescription and told her to get it dispensed at the town chemist shop.

She whined, 'I ain't got naebody t'git it.'

I gestured towards the grubby old character at the other end of the table and said impatiently, 'Get your husband to go.'

Without looking up he muttered, 'Ah'm 'er son,' and continued rolling his fags.

TWENTY YEARS PASSED; I HAD LONG SINCE SWAPPED general practice for specialist medicine. After years of postgraduate training, passing stiff exams, publishing papers in medical journals, and about seven years as a consultant in the air force I was appointed to what I regard as the pinnacle of my medical career, I was Chief of Gastroenterology at the King Faisal Specialist Hospital and Research Centre in Riyadh, the capital of the Kingdom of Saudi Arabia.

This prestigious Royal Hospital had been built on land donated by King Faisal in 1970. It was His Majesty's ambition to build a hospital with specialist services of such a high standard that Saudis would no longer need to travel abroad to obtain medical treatment of international standard. It didn't work out that way – rich Saudis with their retinues continued to travel to centres in London and the United States to enjoy not only excellent medical care but also as an excuse to escape the harsh Saudi climate... cultural as well as physical.

In a macabre turn of events King Faisal might have been the very first patient in his own hospital. On 25 March 1975, some weeks before its official opening, King Faisal was admitted with bullet wounds to the head and died shortly after. He had been shot by a nephew, Prince Faisal bin Mohammad, allegedly crazed by drugs and evil western influences. The prince was beheaded in a public square (Chop Chop Square, Riyadh) on 18 June 1975. The hospital was opened three months later, in September 1975, by King Faisal's successor, King Khalid, and after a further three years I arrived, at first on temporary duty and then in six months invited to return and join the permanent staff.

I spent five years there and left with scores of, mostly happy, memories. One, I remember particularly well, happened in my outpatient clinic. At eight in the morning I strode into my consulting suite and there sitting cross-legged on the examination couch was my first patient, a little, old, wizened Bedouin lady, her face covered in faded blue tattoos and the tip of her nose dyed purple from the lining of her burqa, her face mask. Her sparse hair was generously hennaed and of a startling orange colour. She was not wearing her all-enveloping black abaya cloak and her beak-like face mask; she was dressed only in a tie-at-the-back, pale-blue hospital examination gown.

She looked up, saw me and, horrified, pulled the examination gown up to cover her face – Al'hamdulillah (Thank God) she had managed to quickly cover her exposed face in front of this infidel westerner, this kafir – but below her neck she was stark naked. Although fleeting, the picture is permanently engraved on my memory. To this day it remains as vivid as it was then, even though I caught only a glimpse – a squatting, naked, scrawny, wrinkled old Bedu lady, breasts like two fried eggs with remarkably large, proud, projecting jet-black nipples, perched cross-legged on the examination couch and holding a pale blue examination gown on fully extended arms high above her head.

The Lebanese nurse-interpreter acted swiftly; keeping the old lady's face covered she lay her down and covered her with a sheet. Through that Lebanese nurse-interpreter I took a history, examined the patient and sent her for blood tests and a scan. Then I turned to the nurse and asked her to send in the next patient.

WHAT A CONTRAST! IN SWEPT ONE OF THE MOST STUNNING BEAUTIES I had ever seen. She arrived, unmasked, on a gust of expensive, exotic perfume. Her notes said she was forty-four but she looked twenty-four and with her kohl-rimmed, doe-shaped, black eyes, perfect figure, and generously painted lips she looked like a suicide bomber's promise of paradise. She swept her black cloak around her as she sat down crossing her legs and revealing a tantalising glimpse of a black-stocking clad knee. She sat close to my desk, leaned towards me, smiled a heart-stopping smile and said in a husky, English-girls-public-school-voice, 'Good morning, doctor.'

She was closely followed by her male escort, a Saudi dressed in an impeccably laundered white robe, a thobe, which reached down to his Gucci sandals. He had a red and white check goutra on his head; sported a gold watch as thin as a postage stamp and gold cuff-links, each weighing about an ounce. He too was densely perfumed; she motioned him to sit next to her.

She had a difficult problem. Her doctor's referral letter told me that she had well-established, but compensated, chronic liver disease and she had been referred to me for advice concerning contraception. Were oral contraceptives out because of her liver problem? They were, and in taking her history I soon established that she did not want tubal ligation or any mechanical device. The nurse took her to the examination room, and while the nurse was preparing her for examination I took the opportunity to discuss the situation with her husband, who also had impeccable English.

I told him that as far as I could see the only alternative was that he should undergo vasectomy; a small operation to tie his spermatic cords and render him infertile. I explained this very gently; Saudi males don't go for that sort of thing.

Not surprisingly he became agitated. As the discussion continued he became more and more agitated – finally he got up; he paced the room, up and down, up and down, muttering, 'Why me? Why Me...?'

Finally he turned, faced me and exclaimed, 'But why me, doctor? I'm her son.'

8. SAUDI ARABIA – MY FIRST GLIMPSE OF THE MAGIC KINGDOM

SIX HOURS OUTBOUND FROM LONDON HEATHROW the Lockheed Tristar, in the dark green livery of Saudi Arabian Airlines, gently banked as it joined the circuit over Riyadh. The movement barely registered in first class as I sat sipping 'Saudi Champagne' – apple juice and fizzy water – from a crystal flute.

It was one in the morning, local time. For the past two hours the view from the cabin window had been a uniform jet black as we overflew the vast empty spaces that make up most of the Kingdom of Saudi Arabia. Suddenly myriad twinkling lights appeared below and, as we descended, villas and palaces could be distinguished, each festooned with fairground lights; the streets were crowded with speeding cars, and swirling dust devils obscured patches of the panorama below.

Immediately after the aircraft touched down, the intercom broke into agitated Arabic, to me a harsh unfamiliar guttural language, punctuated by clicks, groans, and glottal strangulations. Then, in English, it welcomed us to Riyadh, told us the local time, that the outside temperature was twenty-two degrees Celsius and that we must remain in our seats until the aircraft came to a complete stop.

Complete stop? I remember at the time thinking to myself, what's an incomplete stop?

The instruction to remain seated did not apply to all passengers... the Saudis as one, got up, wrenched their cases out of the overhead lockers and as they jostled towards the front exit, pushed aside the open-mouthed, impotent Lebanese air hostesses. That was my first encounter with the soon-to-be-familiar basic law that in their Magical Kingdom, Saudis come first, do not need to follow the rules, and can do as they please.

My first of many flights on Saudi Arabian Airlines had been, from the beginning, a strange experience. To start with, at Heathrow a number of attractive, young, and slender Saudi girls trooped aboard. Each was dressed in designer jeans, designer belts and designer shoes. All were dripping in gold and sported standard-issue, gold, bejewelled Rolex watches. An hour before we were due to land at Riyadh these princesses of Arabia disappeared, one-by-one.

Carrying Gucci vanity cases, these flowers of the desert, or more appropriately, offspring of oil, made their way to the toilets. After a few minutes, again, one-by-one, they emerged transformed. Now they were totally in black; all wore abayas, the black all-enveloping cloaks. Their trendy hair styles were covered with black scarves and a few were wearing black burqas, face masks. Meanwhile their brothers, fathers, or husbands (Saudi women, to this day, are not allowed to travel without being escorted by a male family member) remained dozing in their seats, clad in their Savile Row suits and Jermyn Street shirts.

We landed with scarcely a tremor and deplaned into air-conditioned buses for the short drive to the Arrivals Lounge where we were divided into Saudis, Europeans and others. My bags were searched diligently by a young bearded customs officer with an irritating sniff and a suspicious eye. He went over my belongings like a forensic scientist investigating a murder. At last, with a cry, 'Yallah!' He came upon the only vile pornographic material I was carrying. It was in a copy of Punch, a magazine, innocent, humorous, satirical, and sadly now, defunct for many years. I had bought it at Heathrow, on the inside of the back cover was a photograph displaying an advertisement by Kodak. The advert was for 35 millimetre film and showed attractive western maidens, in one-piece bathing costumes, lounging around the rippling blue waters of a swimming pool.

'Ah! Ha!' He cried triumphantly, having unearthed one more evil person entering his sin-free, sacred kingdom. He turned to me; sanctimoniously raised his eyes, fixed me with a disapproving stare and said, 'This is bad things. This is very bad things! You know you coming into the Kingdom of Holy Places and such badness is not allowed.'

With that, with his left thumb he scrunched the advert, tore it out and dropped it on the floor, stood on it, ground it with his heel, glared at me, and said, 'For this I could send you to prison but Allah kareem (God is generous), I will not, but next time I will.'

With a flourish he chalked my bags. I picked them up and left through the Arrivals Exit wondering if I had done the right thing in coming to work for a month as a locum tenens gastroenterologist in this bizarre country. My initial experiences with the Saudis on the aircraft and in the Customs Hall of the airport had left me wondering... more was to come.

Amid the mob, crowding the exit gates, I spotted a young Saudi dressed in a red and white check head dress and a brilliantly starched white thobe holding a large sign which read, 'DOCTOR LARK.' I introduced myself, he told me he was called Mohammed and he allowed me to struggle with my bags to a large American limousine waiting outside.

His English was pretty good and he wasted no time in telling me that normally he didn't do driving but that he was here tonight to do me a special favour. As his English was so unexpectedly fluent I engaged in conversation with him hoping to pick up nuggets of information about this Magical Kingdom which I had just entered. He didn't seem particularly keen to talk until suddenly he asked, 'How old are you?'

'Forty-five,' I replied.

Bluntly he demanded, 'Can you still get it up?'

Stunned, I considered how I would reply, but almost immediately, he went on, 'You are old, very old, and you are not young like me. I am wonderful with the ladies, very wonderful, they all love me. I love them too, especially Egyptian girls, they know all about making love, Filipinas is good too, but your English and your American womens is just silly.'

He became silent, ruminating no doubt on his good fortune at being such a great Saudi stallion and what might be waiting for him after he had dropped me at the end of the journey. I also lapsed into silence and briefly thanked him when he drove me, at four in the morning, into a large, sleeping, compound. He deposited me at the door of the small two-up, two-down house in which I was to live for the next four weeks. As I climbed the stairs I heard a gentle snore... I wasn't alone, I would be sharing the accommodation.

Too excited to sleep more than two or three hours I was up early, anxious to see what delights the day had in store. I met my companion. He was Mike Franklin, an Ear, Nose and Throat surgeon. He told me he was doing his third locum at the King Faisal Specialist Hospital, so he knew the ropes, and as we shared a pot of freshly brewed coffee, he gave me a lot of useful advice.

I reported at nine to the hospital reception and was directed to what was called the Amenities Center for orientation. It was a large building, a recreation centre with a small library, pool room, a hall, and an Olympic size swimming pool. Squash courts with stone floors and tennis courts were nearby. There was everything a person could desire with the exception of the equivalent of a medical students' bar.

I joined a group of a dozen new arrivals and a tall, bronzed, slim, young American lady, sporting at least half a dozen clanking gold bangles on each arm began a well-rehearsed address. 'You are all very privileged to have the privilege of working in this very wonderful Kingdom!' She paused. 'Y'all will be privileged to have excellent accommodations, excellent restaurants and have the privilege of meeting our wonderful Saudi Arabian hosts.

'While you are privileged to be here you must remember to obey all the Saudi rules and codes of behaviour. You must dress modestly and males mustn't wear shorts in public [I later learned that Saudi men are turned on by the sight of male thighs] and you must treat our hosts at all times with respect.'

She did not warn us against imitating our gentle hosts in their deep, public nose-probing, energetic genital scratching and lewd staring at western women. In truth, for us there was no great incentive to ogle the local ladies; they mostly appeared as black blobs... but there were one or two on whom a carefully draped black abaya emphasised a seductive figure, and kohl-bedecked eyes hinted at transports of delight.

After a conducted tour of the hospital administration departments we ended up in the Medical Records Department where a lady of uncertain years and a mask-like face, evidence of repeated and not particularly successful plastic surgery, guided us through the complexities of recording clinical notes and dictating letters.

Then she proudly displayed the hospital's computer. Although not so very long ago those were early days in computing. The computer occupied a large air-conditioned, dust-free room. Its guts were visible in a number of free-standing glass fronted cabinets in which large spools whirled. She explained the various uses the hospital was making of the computer and that the King Faisal Hospital was one of the first 'institooshuns' in the world to be 'compooterised.' It was impressive but it took up an awful lot of space.

'Perhaps one day computers will be made smaller,' she added. I imagine that the desktop model I am now sitting at could do at least twice as much and at ten times the speed of the first King Faisal Specialist Hospital computer.

Later that day I met the Chairman of the Department of Medicine, Dr Smithson, an American dermatologist. Short, somehow penguin-like, he was affable and instantly likeable. After a brief description of the department he handed me over to a senior resident to give me a conducted tour of the hospital. In a couple of hours this pleasant young Syrian doctor took me around all the departments of the hospital. I met the chiefs of various services and inspected the vast ultra-modern laboratory. The department of radiology was enormous, including three CT scanners, ultra-sound and radio-isotope departments.

The surgical theatre suite consisted of five operating theatres, four in operation and one held in reserve. The medical library was huge, contained thousands of books and journals. The whole of the medical knowledge of the twentieth century appeared to be available and librarians were at hand to assist in searches. The library floor was deeply carpeted and its ceiling covered in twenty-four-carat gold leaf.

BUT THERE WAS NO ENDOSCOPY UNIT. Contracted for a month as a consultant gastroenterologist I was alarmed; how could I function properly without endoscopes? Eventually one was found at the back of a shelf in one of the operating theatres. I inspected it and found it to be a side-viewing duodenoscope which in my experience had only one use, to enable one to introduce a thin catheter into the bile and pancreatic ducts to carry out special examinations of the biliary system and the pancreas.

There was no alternative; I had to use that instrument for all routine examinations of the upper gastro-intestinal tract. Routinely one used a forward-viewing 'scope to look ahead while proceeding down the oesophagus into the stomach which one would then inflate with air in order to inspect what amounted to the inside of a balloon. Using a forward-viewing scope could be likened to entering the doorway of a room and looking around, but a side-viewing scope would mean I had to slide through the doorway and inspect the room by moving sideways with my nose just a few inches from the surface of the walls, ceiling and floor.

Another 'scope was found, it was a colonoscope, one of the very first models, I had become accustomed to the modern models. Nonetheless, I was able to carry out full examinations of the colon and in a couple of cases demonstrated ulceration caused by tuberculosis in its most distant part, the caecum. By chance a bronchoscope was found at the back of a shelf. This is a very narrow endoscope which can be passed through the nose and down into the lungs via the trachea and bronchi. Transnasal bronchoscopy requires considerable skill and I had mastered the technique at the Brompton Hospital in London. Alas, there was no way I could use this bronchoscope, in placing it in a perforated metal container for gas sterilization, some incredibly careless person had trapped its tip between the edges of the box... all its optical fibres were broken.

I enjoyed the clinical work in my month's locum. I encountered a number of exotic cases in addition to a multitude of run-of-the-mill tumours, ulcers, and inflammatory conditions. The standards were high. Daily ward rounds were conducted by expert clinicians from around the world, mostly from university hospitals in the United States. Teaching junior doctors was important and a pleasure, they were mostly from the Middle East and keen as mustard. A handful of young Saudi doctors were the forerunners of the not-so-distant day when the hospital would be staffed entirely by Saudis.

There was more to the locum than just the hospital experience. I had a couple of fascinating trips to the desert, camping overnight on one – on that occasion I saw for the first time the wonders of the night sky in Saudi Arabia. The atmosphere was totally unpolluted and the moon was vast, it appeared so close that I felt I could stretch out my fingers and touch it. With individual craters clearly visible to the naked eye the brilliant white moon filled half the sky. The desert was almost colourless but as brightly lit as with the sun at noon.

In my second week, Mike, my house companion, the ENT surgeon locum, said one morning over breakfast, 'How about a trip to Chop Chop Square on Friday, should be interesting?'

Chop Chop Square, I had heard of it, in the centre of old Riyadh, it was where executions by beheading and limb amputations were carried out with a sword after Friday noon prayers.

He then told me about a hospital employee who had been executed a month ago.

'His crime?' I asked.

'He was this huge Somali guy and he had tried to rape the wife of one of the hospital doctors.'

'That's surely serious,' I allowed, 'but execution is drastic.'

'Not only drastic,' he said, 'there was a certain sardonic humour.' He explained the black humour.

'The Somali had been employed since well before the hospital first opened and was entitled to a month's wages for every year he had worked. That would amount to a nice little sum for his family in Somalia.'

'And the humour?' I asked.

'Well, terminal benefits here are known as Severance

Pay. On the day of execution the condemned was brought first from jail to the hospital accounts department for him to sign a document. In effect, on his way to have his neck severed and his head separated from his body in Chop Chop Square he was required to sign a form to say that he had received his Severance Pay.'

'So, Bill,' he said, 'think about it, should be interesting, we'll need to leave early, one of my British male nurses will take us in his car.'

I gave it a lot of thought; I wasn't too sure that I wanted to have the image of a crude barbaric execution engraved on my brain for the remainder of my life. But the more I thought about it, the more I thought I should go, if only to witness something that the rest of the world condemned and which would surely be stopped within a decade.

FRIDAY MORNING WAS CLEAR, SUNNY AND COOL. We drove to the centre of Riyadh, parked the car some two hundred metres from Chop Chop Square and walked along the crowded streets, past open shops displaying sacks of colourful spices and several shops selling gold – frankincense and myrrh were also on offer. We strolled past a clock tower; the clock face bore Arabic numerals and stood adjacent to the restored Musmak Fort, a national treasure of mud and brick which commemorates the attack and conquest of Riyadh, as the 19th turned into the 20th century, by Saudi Arabia's first king, Abdul Aziz. Also known as Ibn Saud, the father of the Sauds, he had with him a small band of some twenty men but courageously, and by taking them by surprise, they defeated several hundred of the rival Rashidi tribe.

Noon prayers were not yet over when we joined the large throng in the square. Restless crowds were milling around and an ambulance and a couple of police cars, with their lights flashing, were parked near the Grand Mosque. We waited; I was absorbed in my thoughts, was this really where I wanted to be? Did I really want to see a fellow human being have his head lopped off? The people grew restive, prayers ended and a crowd of worshippers streamed from the mosque and added to the congestion. Suddenly, with wailing sirens, the ambulance and police cars drove off. Today's execution had been postponed, the disappointed crowd dispersed. 'Let's go,' said Mike. 'We'll have to try again next week.'

I breathed a sigh of relief and we found our way back to the car. There was to be no next week for me; over the next couple of days I gave the idea further thought and decided not to go, but Mike and his friend went. There was an execution scheduled for that Friday... and this time it happened.

When Mike returned late on that Friday afternoon he was shaken, he was pale and quiet, he spoke barely half-a-dozen words to me that evening. When, on Saturday evening, he was at last able to describe the event I was even more relieved that I had not witnessed such barbarity. Over a fresh pot of coffee Mike told me what had happened.

'We joined the crowd in Chop Chop Square and just as on last Friday the ambulance and police cars rolled up and parked. As before, at the end of Friday prayers, several hundred worshippers streamed out of the mosque and swelled the crowd. Suddenly the police started pushing the crowd around to make a space the size of a tennis court in front of the mosque; we waited while the police held the crowds back.' Mike was silent for a minute but began again. 'I was taken by surprise and shocked when I was seized by an ugly, bearded scraggy, hawk-nosed, muttaween [religious policeman] in a brown cloak, waving a camel stick. He took my elbow in a grip of iron and dragged me to the front of the crowd. I didn't know at the time that the religious police always forced any foreign onlookers they found in the crowd to the front because it was believed that the condemned man could not enter paradise if his last sight on earth was that of an infidel.

Then a nondescript van drove into the cleared area, the back doors opened and out staggered a young man; blindfolded, manacled, and obviously drugged. The van drove off. The young man, he couldn't have been more than in his early twenties, was forced to kneel in the centre of the space which had been cleared.' Mike drank some coffee, gathered his thoughts and continued:

'After the mob had stood in silence, for what seemed an age but was probably only a few minutes, a heavily bearded official emerged from the mosque and read the charges and sentence. Then a huge, jet-black man holding a large scimitar appeared, it seemed from nowhere, behind the kneeling man. With the tip of his scimitar he pricked the condemned man in the lower back, that caused the young man to jerk his head up, the sword flashed and blood spurted, but the big black guy had made a mess of the job. With his neck deeply injured the poor young fellow keeled over moaning pitifully. Assistants rushed to straighten him; the executioner took another swing but still didn't complete the job.

It was awful, it took him another two swings and then the head, by now mercifully separated from the victim's neck, rolled away a couple of inches. Blood was jetting from the root of his neck but in no time it subsided to a trickle and then, and then... to my utter astonishment, what appeared to be a doctor in a white coat with a trademark stethoscope dangling from his neck, descended from the ambulance and approached the headless corpse. He knelt by it and for half a minute felt for a wrist pulse... he then straightened up and officially declared the headless criminal dead.

As one the crowd yelled, "Allahu wa Akbar" (God is the Greatest) and repeated it, rhythmically, over and over. A couple of attendants threw the body and head onto a stretcher, clumsily shoved it into the van and drove off. The police jumped into their cars, the doctor into the ambulance and they all drove off with sirens wailing.'

Mike stopped, it was a few minutes before he could continue and what he then said made me for ever grateful that I had not witnessed such a ghastly display of primitive religious fervour.

'I HAD TO WATCH THE MOST SICKENING END TO THE AFFAIR. It was impossible to get out from the crowd, there was no way – the mob milled round and round the execution site trampling pools of the victim's blood into the sand, to-and-fro, to-and-fro, getting more and more frenzied and all the time chanting, "Allahu wa Akbar."'

Mike was silent for half-an-hour; I sat with him, also in shocked silence, his description was so vivid. For me relief was mixed with my feelings of horror... relief that I had not witnessed this awful barbarity.

On a more pleasant note, my locum had opened my eyes to the magic of the desert and the pleasures of working with brilliant colleagues with interesting clinical material in a country with a new and intriguing culture. True I had found downsides, Chop Chop Square activities; the place of women in Saudi society, religious intolerance and some aspects of Saudi culture – all were disturbing but on balance I had distinctly positive feelings, I knew I could set up a fine gastroenterology unit and perhaps even make a little difference in this young country.

The locum tenens post had been to replace the staff gastroenterologist, who was elderly and on leave, but I was told that he wasn't showing any indication of quitting despite being close to his seventies. I made it clear, to the chairman of the department of medicine, that I wished to return at some time and next day was on the Saudia flight back to London.

9. 'GOOD MORNING, DOCTOR DOGGY!'

JIM DOCHERTY AND I HAD BEEN PALS since we were medical students and that was a long, long time ago. I knew he'd specialised in psychiatry but I had no idea what he'd been up to for the past twenty years until I bumped into him in a gents' natty outfitters in Lincoln, where, coincidentally, we were both having suits made.

We collided as I emerged from a changing room wearing a jacket and trousers held together by temporary threads and criss-crossed with tailor's chalk.

We exclaimed in unison.

'Bill!'

'Jim!'

'What on earth are you doing in Lincoln?'

'I'm in the air force and boss of the medical department at the RAF hospital ten miles from here, and you?'

'Oh, I'm spending two or three days visiting friends while taking a look around the old hospital.'

Delighted to meet Jim, I invited him to dine with me in the Officers' Mess the following evening. Before we ate the craic flowed as easily as the mess bar's best bitter. Jim, now a consultant psychiatrist in one of the London teaching hospitals also had a smart private practice with rooms in Harley Street. As part of his training Jim had worked for four years as a senior registrar at the Lincolnshire County Mental Hospital and explained that he had lately developed a yearning to visit the place and refresh pleasant memories of old friends and the consultants who had trained him.

'And what's your most striking memory?' I asked.

He thought for a moment. 'Funnily enough it's neither old friends nor old teachers, it's a patient I remembered vividly from when I first joined the hospital twenty years ago.'

I was intrigued, 'Tell me more.'

'She was a long-stay patient, sixty years old when I joined the hospital. She was called Lily Perry; we all called her 'Lil'. She was liked by everybody, did no harm, didn't cause any fuss and didn't get in anybody's way because she spent her days walking up and down the long glass corridor between the south and north wings of the hospital. Up and down she'd go, up and down, ceaselessly, endlessly, up and down. She wasn't directly under my care but I had taken a look at her chart, which was years old, dog-eared and had had no entry for six months, and that was when she simply had a cold.' Jim paused, took a draught, and went on:

'Lil had been admitted fifteen years earlier with a life-crippling obsessive compulsive disorder. In addition to washing her hands every few minutes she was compelled to polish all the metallic objects in her house several times a day and she had to pick up spent matches wherever she saw them – easy if at home but if she was on a bus and spotted one on the pavement she had to jump off the bus to pick it up. If she went to a pub she would grub through ash trays to extract grimy matches; if she found herself standing next to a bloke and he lit up she would demand he gave her the spent match. A major social problem with Lil was that she was alone; her husband had left her and her children wanted nothing to do with their nutty mother.'

'Did she respond to treatment?' I asked.

'Well, yes and no,' Jim replied. 'She was given electroconvulsive therapy, intensive counselling, psychotropic drugs, aversion therapy and cognitive behavioural modification.'

I raised a brow and asked, 'And did she improve?'

'As I said, yes and no,' replied Jim. 'She no longer washed her hands dozens of times a day, she no longer picked up matchsticks but she sublimated all her obsessions into walking that long stone-floored corridor. Every day when I worked there and went from ward to ward I'd meet Lil each time, as she went up and down, up and down, and every time she encountered me she would pause, look me in the eye and say, "Good morning, Doctor Doggy" or, "Good afternoon, Doctor Doggy."

'She couldn't get her mind around my name, Docherty; she called me 'Doggy.' So at least twice a day it was, good morning Doctor Doggy, good afternoon Doctor Doggy, or good evening Doctor Doggy.

DURING THE FOUR YEARS I WAS THERE LIL'S HIPS started to play up, and no wonder, they were wearing out. Up and down, up and down that thirty-yard long, unforgiving stone floor, day in day out, month in month out, no time off for any reason. She'd begin promptly after breakfast and break off only for lunch and supper; even then she was compelled at times to abandon a meal mid-way through so that she could resume her walking. Lil was bird-like, slender, neatly dressed with her hair always coiffed. Towards the end of my time there she took to walking with two sticks. Her hips were hurting and walking had become increasingly difficult.

On her bad days she would stagger slowly along like an

insect with a broken leg. But always she paused when we met in the corridor; looked me in the eyes, gave me a smile and cheerily said, "Good morning, Doctor Doggy."'

Jim took another swig of beer and went on. 'When I returned a couple of days ago I was sitting having a coffee with an old colleague and asked him if Lil was still walking the corridor. "Oh, yes," he replied, "but Lil wore out her hips and had both operated on five years ago. Now it looks as though she's wearing out the artificial joints she was given, but yes, she walks the walk as she always did. Mind you, she's now over eighty and she struggles."'

I took a drink of my beer and, plunged in thought, waited for Jim to continue his trip down memory lane.

'The second day I was there I spotted Lil as I wandered around those familiar surroundings; which as far as I could see, hadn't changed at all, even smelled the same, a mixture of disinfectant, floor polish, and stale cabbage. I stopped and watched as she slowly approached me. She hadn't seen me; her back had bent, her eyes were fixed on the floor a yard or so ahead of her feet. Her bony, blue-veined, old hands grasped the handles of a wheeled Zimmer frame as she wobbled slowly along. Time had not spared Lil since I had last seen her fifteen years before. I stood and watched as she approached, head down, shoulders rounded, feet shuffling. Seeing my feet she paused... she raised her head, our eyes met and she smiled gently, "Good morning, Doctor Doggy," she said.'

Jim paused. 'Then she dropped her eyes and shuffled on.' Jim drained his tankard put it down and then said, 'Just think, Bill, all the years we have been frantically working our butts off and forging our careers Lil's been walking that corridor.'

I could see his eyes were moist... and so were mine, with a sigh he said, 'And she's going to do that until she dies.'

10. THE GREAT GAME WILL GO ON AND ON…

'When everyone is dead The Great Game is finished; not before.' Kim – Rudyard Kipling

IT WAS DEEP MID-WINTER, BUT THE MORNING SUN BLAZED through the curtains of the window of my consulting room, the sky was a deep, cloudless blue. Outside it was 22°C, the bulbuls warbled their sweet song and a flock of mynah birds squabbled noisily on the lawn. It hadn't rained for twelve months; this was Dubai.

Sitting opposite, across my desk, a bent, broken, and masked woman, covered from head to toe in black, sobbed. She had been brought to me by Mohammed Shah, a tall, distinguished, silver-haired, clean-shaven Afghan wearing a three piece, navy-blue, pin-stripe suit, and a collarless white shirt closed at the neck with an old-fashioned brass stud.

'Doctor Lark, she very sad,' Mohammed explained.

'She fly from Pakistan yesterday. For seven days she and five childrens walking through snow in very high mountains in Ofgoneestan, one of her childrens is died, her husband is died. Mujahideen say he spy, shoot him in backside of head. She very, very sad and all time she throw up, please you make her better Doctor Lark.'

I took her medical history; for years she had suffered episodes of nasty upper abdominal pain, often waking her in the early hours, sometimes she vomited and that would ease her pain. I examined her; she had localised finger-point tenderness in the upper abdomen. I ordered a blood test. The result was through in twenty minutes – it was positive for an infection with a bacterium called Helicobacter pylori which is associated with ulcers and causes inflammation of the stomach and duodenum. I wrote a prescription and asked her to return in a week.

Mohammed brought her back, she was well, her pain had gone, she was not vomiting and she was pleased. She almost certainly had had an ulcer which would be permanently cured by completing the course of treatment, the very same treatment which I had prescribed for the many Afghans I saw in my practice. It seemed that many Afghans in Dubai had indigestion and every one of them I saw had helicobacter infection. Fortunately for my reputation and practice, all responded nicely to treatment.

Mohammed Shah was a successful business man; the de facto sage and godfather of the large Dubai Afghan community. One day he said to me, 'Doctor Lark, you have nice clinic, I want you make same in Kabul, you be boss.'

'Kabul?' I said. 'It is dangerous there.'

'No, no, Kabul safe, plenty policemens, plenty soldiers.'

I had no intention of going to Kabul… 'But this is a private clinic and there is no money in Kabul.'

He looked at me, astonished. 'No moneys in Kabul? No Doctor Lark there is plenty moneys in Kabul.'

My eyebrows went up, he went on. 'Yes, yes, plenty

moneys – moneys from Amerikee, Canadee, Britannee, Ferrancee, plenty, plenty moneys.'

AND THERE YOU HAVE IT – THE AFGHAN MINDSET. Vast funds donated by other countries to improve Afghanistan's governance and the lot of its people up for grabs... fair game for all Afghans. That conversation took place way before 11 September 2001; plenty, plenty more moneys has poured into Afghanistan since then.

Mohammad's attitude was as sincere and natural to him as it would be to the majority of his thirty-five million fellow Afghans. If you add to that mindset; centuries of inter-tribal conflict, xenophobia, corruption from top to bottom, a country bristling with arms, Islamic extremism in the form of the fanatic Taliban, a prosperous, crooked opium and cannabis agriculture, and a hostile terrain and climate – what do you get?

You get a place to avoid... and at all costs to avoid making war there.

Kipling's 'Great Game' referred to espionage and counter-espionage in the days of the British Raj; to those days when aggressive, armed, savage hill tribes threatened the safety of the Empire in India and three futile wars were fought by the British Army.

In truth, however, the Great Game had started three millennia before. Would-be conquerors, Persians, Mongols, Turks, Arabs, and even Alexander the Great were in turn brought to a stop by fierce tribesmen in what is now Afghanistan. And it was in Afghanistan that the British Army suffered what has been described as its worst ever defeat; a horrible tale beginning with an uprising in Kabul which brought the First Anglo-Afghan war to an abrupt end in 1842.

IN 1839 – ON THE BASIS OF PHONEY INTELLIGENCE that Russia was planning to invade

Afghanistan as a preliminary to an invasion of India – the army of the British Raj invaded Afghanistan and installed a puppet government in Kabul. The British declared that as soon as the Afghan army was capable of defending its own country the army of the Raj would be withdrawn. Meanwhile, the Afghan people should enjoy the pleasures and benefits of the presence of the benign invaders.

Some pleasures! Some benefits! The British officers enjoyed the local dancing girls; they played cricket, hunted boar, drank the fine wines and smoked the two camel-loads of cigars they had brought from India. Already hated, for their un-Islamic ways, the British imposed additional taxes to fund their stay. Resentful tribes, traditionally at loggerheads with each other, united in their loathing of the British.

In November 1841 a senior British officer, lieutenant colonel Sir Alexander Burnes, and his aides, were killed by a mob in Kabul. Quite out of character, the British military took no action. This weakness encouraged further revolt. A month later the British envoy, Sir William Mcnaghten, was seized and beheaded. His dismembered body was displayed on a meat hook in the bazaar and his head, impaled on a stake, was paraded through the streets.

The British contingent in Kabul, now numbering some 5,000 troops and 10,000 camp followers (families and civilian workers), was in disarray. Their leaders negotiated with the Afghan warlords and a few days later, after handing over all its finances and artillery and being reassured by the promise of safe passage from Kabul to Jalalabad, eighty miles to the east, the 15,000 strong British garrison set off.

Shuffling, frozen, starving columns trudged through the January snows. Day after day their numbers diminished as scores were picked off, the easiest of prey for the Afghan tribesmen's muzzle-loading Jezail muskets. In mid-January 1842 the final British square fought to the death and, with any remaining civilians, was slaughtered on a hill near the village of Gandamak, thirty-five miles from Jalalabad.

Only one Englishman survived, he was army surgeon William Brydon. As the wounded Dr Brydon weaved his exhausted way through the gates of Jalalabad, on an even more exhausted pony, a sentry asked him, 'Where's the army?'

Surgeon Brydon replied, 'I am the army.'

After a couple of yards the pony collapsed and was dead before it hit the ground.

Again, and yet again, on the basis of imminent invasion of Afghanistan by Russia seeking access to the Indian Ocean, the British Raj fought another two Anglo-Afghan wars, each with no lasting success.

In 1979 the mighty Russian army entered Afghanistan to restore order at the invitation of the government. Tribal unrest and a guerrilla organisation, in the form of the Mujahideen, threatened the legitimate regime. A decade later, in 1989, the mighty Soviet army retreated with its tail between its legs. That modern army was no match for the ragtag guerrillas of the Mujahideen.

THERE HAVE BEEN TWO EPOCHAL ATTACKS ON THE MIGHT OF UNCLE SAM; both were destined to forever change the face of the world. The first, the Japanese attack on Pearl Harbour on 7 December 1942 which precipitated the entry of America into World War II. The second, terrorist air attacks using hijacked civil airliners as surrogate suicide bombs on 11 September 2001. Flown by terrorists associated with al-Qaeda the aircraft were flown into New York skyscrapers, the Twin Towers of the World Trade Centre, and into the Pentagon, the headquarters of the American military in Arlington, Virginia. Very nearly three thousand people were killed that day... which has become known for all eternity as 'nine eleven' – '9/11.'

When, to avenge 9/11, US President George Bush led

the invasion of Afghanistan on 10/7 (7 October 2001) he promised the American people he would seek out and destroy the terrorists and those who were sheltering them. One could be forgiven for imagining that Mr Bush would think that with the military might of the United States, and her Allies, the guerrilla rabble of the Islamic extremists, the Taliban, would be easy pickings and dealt with within a matter of weeks or months while at the same time al-Qaeda and its leader, Osama bin Laden, would be no more.

But no, Operation 'Enduring Freedom,' as Bush called his invasion, proved to be more of an enduring than a freeing exercise. The many times repeated pattern was that as the Allies took control of an Afghan village the guerrillas would melt away – only to creep back when the allied forces moved elsewhere.

It is staggering to think that by the time the Allied combat forces left Afghanistan at the end of 2014 they had spent fourteen years in a vain effort to attempt to win a war against a guerrilla army. Why staggering? Because it took only six years for those same Allies to defeat the mighty military empires of Japan and Nazi Germany in World War II (September 1939 to August 1945). The real tragedy is that, despite the rhetoric, the Allies have never been much closer to victory than George Bush was on the very first day he set foot in Afghanistan.

True, the Americans achieved a coup when US Navy Seals assassinated Osama bin Laden in May 2011. Alas, this achievement was tarnished a few months later by a Taliban, with a hand-held, rocket-propelled grenade launcher resting on his shoulder, shooting down a Chinook helicopter and killing all thirty-eight on board… of which twenty-two were Navy Seals.

The Allies devoted vast sums of money and effort to train Afghan police and military forces in order to ensure peace in the country once the international forces left. But will peace follow after the withdrawal of Allied combat forces? Events have shown that insurgents easily infiltrate the police and the Afghan army. Afghan individual loyalty has always proved impossible to monitor. Thousands of assassinations have been carried out by uniformed members of the Afghan security forces in attacks euphemistically called Green on Blue. It was the young men from the West who had borne the brunt of Green on Blue attacks. Those attacks were impossible to predict as they were invariably surprise attacks carried out either by genuine uniformed Afghan police or military with records of years of loyal service who had clandestinely joined the insurgents, or attacks carried out by Taliban disguised in army or police uniforms bought for a few dollars in local bazaars.

In 2012, one in five deaths in NATO personnel occurred as a result of Green on Blue attacks, young men were shot dead by an Afghan 'ally.' Insurgents and ordinary civilians were indistinguishable... the man scratching around in a field could have been a farmer trying to get carrots to grow in the inhospitable terrain, or equally he might have been an insurgent planting an IED (Improvised Explosive Device).

AND HOW WELL DID THE AFGHANS RESPOND to training? Poorly, if a mass escape of Taliban prisoners from Khandahar jail is anything to go by. Insurgents had dug a tunnel an incredible one kilometre long from a workshop outside the jail. It passed under a main road and ended deep inside the jail. The tunnel was well constructed; electricity pilfered from the local supply provided lighting and fans were installed to ensure a circulation of fresh air. It was reported that 546 prisoners escaped in one night, unnoticed. Unnoticed? Because as one recaptured escapee said, 'All the guards were sleeping; they had had their evening marijuana and heroin.'

It is delusional to suppose that after the Allies eventually withdraw residual 'peacekeeping' forces that

Afghanistan will become a tranquil self-governing country with its own reliable security services and its citizens going about their daily lives as freely as their counterparts in the West. The West will forever ignore the centuries of Afghan history of rampant corruption, bribery, assassinations and treachery.

Concerns about what will happen in Afghanistan, when Allied forces totally withdraw, are echoed by a retired Afghan military spokesman who predicts that chaos and inter-factional conflict will reign. After the Allies leave, Afghanistan will revert to its old ways; maybe not immediately, or in a year, or in a decade; but the odds are that it will happen, as it has time and time again over three millennia.

What is the legacy of the Allies? What have the Allies achieved? 'Nothing,' according to Mohammed Karzai, ex-President of Afghanistan. When he spoke in early 2014, with just six months remaining of his presidency, he said, 'On the security front the entire NATO exercise was one that caused Afghanistan a lot of suffering, a lot of loss of life, and no gains, because the country is not secure. NATO incorrectly focussed the fight on Afghan villages rather than attacking Taliban havens in Pakistan.'

Can there be any doubt that Afghanistan will revert to its pre-Bush-invasion state? In August 2016 the government in Kabul reported that it had lost a further 5% of the country's territory since the beginning of the year – that meant that the Taliban already controlled one third of Afghanistan. The United Nations reported that, in that same period, 5,166 people (a third children) had been killed or injured

The West must get out and not wait for the ultimate end predicted by Kipling's character in Kim, Hurree Babu: 'The Great Game is over when everyone is dead. Not before.' Is it too much to hope that future leaders in the West will learn the lessons taught by recent and ancient history… never, never, invade Afghanistan??

11. MOTHER NATURE, IS SHE A GOOD PARENT?

WHEN I WAS A MEDICAL STUDENT I SPENT HOUR after hour gazing down microscopes and was always amazed by the complexity and the beauty of the minutiae of the living world. And when it came to studying how plants and animals function, I was equally astonished. Repeatedly I would ask myself what supremely intelligent force could produce such diverse, beautiful, complicated structures and ensure that they functioned year-in-year-out. For the religious there is a ready explanation but for others there is no simple answer, in fact, there is no answer.

Since time immemorial man has puzzled over the nature of his world and the nature of his existence, a philosophy which is called Cosmology, and which in recent decades, because of the development of various hypotheses, is now called Scientific Cosmology. Rationalists say that it was out of humanity's need for answers that the world's religions appeared – while those of religious persuasion maintain that divine revelations form the basis of their faith, their belief in God, and in how the universe was created.

In 1193 the Archbishop of Canterbury, St Anselm, defined God as, '*something greater than which nothing can be conceived.*' The archbishop thought that this statement standing alone, by itself, was proof of the very existence of God. Eight centuries later, after years of occasionally thinking about the Archbishop's words, the British philosopher, Lord Bertrand Russell, related that he was in a newsagent's shop buying a copy of The Times of London when he experienced an epiphany, a flash of insight, and to his surprise found that he totally agreed with the Archbishop.

Throughout the ages cosmologists have questioned and studied the origins of the universe; but despite legends and theories, Big Bangs and Black Holes, the answer remains elusive. Another premise, the Design Argument, puts it in a deceptively simple sentence... Because the world is ordered, God must exist.

The truth is that we don't know. Even that militant atheist Richard Dawkins ducked the issue by defining himself as an agnostic atheist – which would appear to translate as an unknowing, disbeliever in God.

If we accept that every aspect of what we might call Mother Nature was created by, *something greater than which anything can be conceived,* we can then study her without the fruitless mental torment of trying to define her creator. We can study how she impacts our lives and we can study how we interact with her. We regard Mother Nature as the guardian of our health and a major part of the study of medicine is to understand how she works on our behalf. Things go wrong at times and then, hopefully, doctors can step in to help her combat disease, mend broken limbs and slow the ravages of old age.

From the days of Hippocrates to the Age of Enlightenment physicians practised their healing art without much rational basis and according to various, mainly non-scientific, systems – Greek and Arabic for the most part. In the dark ages of medicine doctors had lacked scientific knowledge and had no appreciation of the harm they were unwittingly inflicting. The dawn of the age of medical enlightenment broke with William Harvey's description of the circulatory system; but it wasn't until the mid-nineteenth century, with the coming of anaesthesia and knowledge of the transmission of infections, that the light truly shone.

Up to that time the medical profession was divided into physicians and surgeons and both had alarming (unpublished) mortality rates. Only the lucky survived the surgeon's swift, cut, tie, and cauterize operations. Physicians took a more leisurely pace to kill more than they cured. Their medicaments were directed towards giving the patient severe diarrhoea with purgatives, making him vomit with emetics, giving him herbal medications with fanciful curative properties and toxic medications containing arsenic or mercury. For centuries conventional treatments included; bleeding by opening a vein in the arm, applying poultices of various substances including bread and linseed, blistering the skin with heated cups, applying blood-sucking leeches and not least, squirting healing liquids through a big, fearsome, metal syringe, called a clyster, inserted into the rectum – even tobacco smoke was injected with bellows in the belief that it exerted a therapeutic effect.

HOWEVER THERE WAS AN AUSTRIAN PHYSICIAN whose treatments were totally free from harmful effects and because of that he met with great success and his methods became popular. His preparations were no more toxic than a glass of water.

His method was to dilute what he called the active substance of his medications to such an extent that it could no longer be detected in solution. He then administered what was in effect water, with a good dose of medical propaganda. To this day, despite no convincing evidence of anything other than placebo effect, his system has millions of adherents, including members of the British Royal family and a handful of properly qualified but misguided doctors.

That Austrian physician was Dr Samuel Hahnemann (1755-1843), and he called his method of treatment 'Homeopathy'. In truth he was simply following the dictum drummed into the head of every medical student: *primum non nocere*, first do no harm.

Hahnemann did not discover homeopathy in the way that Fleming discovered penicillin, he invented it.

In Hahnemann's time, conventional physicians killed in droves, but Hahnemann's homeopathy did no harm. Unconsciously, simply by allowing Mother Nature a free rein, and by itself being totally free of side effects, the ascent of homeopathy was guaranteed. Nature did her business – Hahnemann took the credit – homeopathy's reputation was established.

With the medical advances of the past century man's ability to fight disease has increased exponentially, but not always with safety. It might appear that, aside from trauma, patients get admitted to hospital because Mother Nature has slipped up somewhere, or has she? In a significant number it is the doctor who has slipped up; then we call the illness iatrogenic – caused by the iatros (Greek for physician). Otherwise illnesses are attributable to what can be described as natural causes. Has Mother Nature made a mistake? Are infections like malaria, bubonic plague, poliomyelitis, typhus, or measles all the result of accidents in nature?

Mother Nature looks after countless species and her duty is the same to each... survival of that species, even though one particular species may cause a disease in another. An endless cycle of infection-transmission-infection-transmission ensures species continuation in infectious diseases. The plasmodium parasites of malaria, the bacteria of the plague, and the viruses of influenza continue their existence by being passed from host to host by well-established means. Mosquitoes transmit malaria, rat fleas pass on the plague, while for viruses, airborne aerosols produced by coughing or sneezing, and surface contamination provide media for transmission.

Mother Nature provides her species with defence mechanisms. Humans have white blood cells and immune systems to fight infections. The young are better at combating infection than the old; equally the young are best at reproduction. Mother Nature does not have a lot of time for oldies. She allows them to age, to degenerate, to develop cancers and have strokes, and heart attacks.

Oldies no longer reproduce, they aren't much good at hunting and gathering, so she demonstrates their uselessness to potential mates by the appearance of lines on their faces, wrinkles everywhere, hairs growing out of men's ears and noses, lady's breasts drooping alarmingly, hair turning grey, if it hasn't already fallen out – all signs that an individual's reproductive life is over – Mother Nature has little interest in the old for species survival. It has to be admitted, however, that in the distant past the older members of human tribes possessed a hoard of useful experiences which could be passed on and help tribal survival. In the end it is the individual who is most interested in longevity, and as life-expectation increases, mainly because of vast improvements in hygiene, the anti-ageing industry expands.

There are examples in which man has taken on and won against some of Mother Nature's species which are dangerous to him. He has eradicated smallpox by vaccination, reduced malaria by draining swamps and cholera outbreaks occur when community hygiene breaks down. Poliomyelitis would almost certainly by now be extinct but for religious extremists in primitive communities spreading rumours that the polio vaccine causes sterility, or that the teams of charitable workers administering the vaccine are spies for the Satanic West. Man has been successful in prolonging human lifespan by decades, by being able to treat most killer infectious diseases, and by massive improvements in hygiene. Horse manure no longer decorates city streets, public sanitation provides clean drinking water, and sewage systems hygienically dispose of infective human waste.

Mother Nature has some intriguing tricks up her sleeve to promote individual species survival. Take for example her use of fleas on the backs of rats to promote survival of the plague bacillus. Rat fleas infected with the plague bacillus cannot swallow; their swallowing mechanism is paralysed by a toxin made by the plague bacillus. An inability to swallow makes the fleas frantic for their usual sustenance, blood, and when the plague-ridden host, usually the rat, dies, they hop off to look for that sustenance elsewhere – human blood serves them equally well. The plague bacilli take up residence in the flea's stomach in a clot of blood which the flea is unable to digest. A small amount of the plague-infected clot is regurgitated into the victim when bitten by the flea. The plague disease vectors, fleas, rats, and humans die, but the plague species continues.

Another example of Mother Nature's genius for manipulation and ensuring species survival also involves the rat. The survival of the species Mother Nature is concerned with this time is a humble single-celled organism called Toxoplasma gondii. Incredibly, in this example, Mother Nature artfully makes male rats fall in love with cats. Normally when a male rat catches a whiff of the scent of a cat he runs like the wind, but toxoplasma has a cunning mechanism for causing a fatal feline attraction.

WHEN A MALE RAT SWALLOWS SOMETHING CONTAMINATED with toxoplasma cysts the capsules of the cysts are digested releasing the tiny parasites which enter the rat's blood stream through the wall of the intestine. The tiny forms of toxoplasma circulate in the rat's blood and settle in that part of the rat's brain concerned with sexual attraction; that part which lights up when Mr Rat sees or scents an attractive lady rat. However, when that part of Mr Rat's brain has been colonized by toxoplasma it develops a totally different agenda. If toxoplasma-infected Mr Rat sniffs out a cat in the vicinity he no longer tears away, he dashes towards the alluring pussy; the cat kills and eats him and a new cycle for toxoplasma propagation begins.

It is one of nature's basic laws that sexual reproduction is essential for species rejuvenation and survival. Toxoplasma can only reproduce sexually in one place, a cat's small intestine. In the cat's small intestine the toxoplasma become intensely active and sexual reproduction results in the primary host, the cat, excreting ten million oöcysts (eggs) a day. These cysts have tough capsules and remain viable for years in dirt, on plants or in the soil. The hardy cysts hang around in their billions until they are swallowed by a rat, mouse, bird, or other warm blooded creature which cats like to eat. Humans pick up the cysts by direct contact with toxoplasma carrying cats and from cat litter. Toxoplasma cysts are everywhere, they are ingested by eating unwashed fruit and vegetables, eating raw meat and lamb when it is – especially the way the French like it – an under-cooked pink. No apparent harm is done to humans unless the human happens to be a pregnant woman or has an immune deficiency secondary to, for example, cancer or AIDS.

There is an interesting spin-off from the discovery of the origin of this perversion of rat behaviour. It has been suggested that the conundrum of the causation of schizophrenia, which still baffles medical science, may be triggered by toxoplasma infection in humans. Thus far it has been shown that schizophrenics have a somewhat higher incidence of positive blood tests for toxoplasmosis and that the drugs which dampen down schizophrenic behaviour will have the effect of reducing infected rats' attraction to cats. Research has a long way to go but it is just possible that there is a link between the mechanism of rats falling in love with cats and schizophrenia.

Perhaps toxoplasmosis could be implicated in the formation of brain tumours or behaviour disorders like hyperactivity associated with attention deficit. There is some evidence that toxoplasma may be associated with changes in human behaviour. Women infected with toxoplasma are more likely to stray from the marital fold and infected men may become more aggressive.

Yet another example of manipulative Mother Nature occurs in the world of amphibians. There has been a dramatic and worldwide decline in populations of amphibians in recent years. This has been caused by two phenomena. First: man-made changes to amphibians' environment, draining wetlands and ponds and pouring toxic industrial wastes into rivers. Second: Mother Nature up to her tricks again, scientists have observed in recent years that vast numbers with deformed and extra limbs have appeared in local amphibian populations. These handicapped individuals are less able to escape wading birds, their natural predators. This startling effect ensures the survival of a tiny flat worm, Ribeiroia ondatrae. This worm parasite reproduces asexually inside aquatic snails which release thousands of infectious larvae which burrow into the developing limb buds of various amphibians.

In tadpoles they cause the formation of deformed or extra limbs as they mature into frogs. Not as nimble as they should be, those frogs make easy prey for predatory water birds. When a heron swallows and digests the deformed amphibian, larvae are released into in the bird's intestines where sexual reproduction takes place and thousands of egg-cysts are released back into the water where they are eaten by snails, and so the cycle continues.

HAVING GOT THUS FAR YOU MIGHT by now be beginning to wonder what Mother Nature looks like. Is she a charming little old lady with candy in her handbag for good children? Is she Saturn's daughter, Ceres, the Earth Mother, the source of nurturing, patience and unconditional love? Or, could she be like one of Shakespeare's warty witches, prancing and babbling around a bubbling cauldron?

None of these; she looks like a spiral staircase with hand rails on both sides of the stairs which are bent in a double helix. The rails are made of sugarphosphate and the stairs made of bases (nucleotides). The whole makes the foundation of life, the genetic material called DNA (deoxyribonucleic acid).

Where did DNA come from and how old is it? Life came from a primitive soup, or as Charles Darwin called it, a warm little pond. This version of the story of the beginning of life suggests that four billion years ago, the water of the seas contained no living material, while the atmosphere above contained the chemicals, methane, ammonia and hydrogen. Lightning strikes caused the chemicals to combine and amino acids were formed and were deposited in the primordial sea. These chemical compounds became more and more complicated and developed the power to reproduce, to replicate. From then on, it was a question of the evolution of chemical substances of greater and greater complexity until one day DNA popped up.

Is this all totally conjectural? Not at all: in 1952 a twenty-two year old PhD science student called Stanley Miller at the University of Chicago carried out an experiment. He set up apparatus which allowed him to heat water in a flask from which steam passed upwards into another flask which already held a mixture of methane, ammonia and hydrogen (no oxygen) creating the conditions that were thought to exist those four billion years ago. He imitated lightning strikes by having electrodes project into the atmosphere in the upper flask and between them passed a continuous arc of electric current. A week later the liquid in the lower flask had turned brown and contained thirteen of the fourteen amino acids essential to life. Then in 1961 a Spanish scientist showed that amino acids could be made using hydrogen cyanide and he was experimentally able to produce adenine, one of the essential components of DNA.

So is this what happened in the primordial soup with the eventual formation of DNA? But who put the water in Charles Darwin's little warm pond? And where did the hydrogen and oxygen to make the water come from?

Did some sort of living blob appear which evolved from the most primitive life form, bacteria, over millions of years? And then over a few more millions of years further evolve into a living fish-like creature that eventually developed lungs and limbs and at last was able to heave itself out of the water? Over millions upon millions of years that primitive creature developed along different lines and differentiated into the thousands of living species which over the aeons were modified according to Darwin's Laws of Natural Selection. Then Professor Dawkins steps up to the mark and takes over explaining further development on the basis of genetics.

But it's the bit at the very beginning which bothers me, who or what made that primordial soup? Who selected those particular gases and put them in the atmosphere? Some believe that life on earth began with materials that arrived from outer space – that's the Panspermia theory, some proof of which was adduced when a meteorite, which landed in Australia in 1962, was found to be rich in amino acids. But again, for me, Panspermia begs the fundamental question… how did it begin out there?

Jump forward to the present and take, for example, the genetic basis of toxoplasma making rats love cats. The DNA coding providing the instructions necessary to continue the cycle resides inside the nuclei of the oöcysts deposited by the cat. We have seen that these egg cysts hang about on fruit, vegetables, on the cat's fur or in cat litter or on the soil. The secondary host – rat, pig, lamb, or human – inadvertently swallows the cysts which rupture in the intestine releasing a microscopic creature, in length about a tenth the diameter of a human hair. The microscopic creature holds all the toxoplasma's DNA coded genetic material which has been transmitted through every stage of its life-cycle. This tiny thing, called a tachyzoite, is programmed to penetrate the host's intestinal wall, enter the bloodstream and end up in nerve or muscle tissue. It is directed to the 'love centre' of the brain of the male rat by the coding of the DNA – but who did all that? Who, or what, put that coding there? It's all very well to say a mutation generated the code but how did the mechanism of directing the tachyzoite develop, at random, by a billion to one chance? How did it work out which part of the male rat's brain to settle in?

It has to be accepted that there are no fundamental explanations for the many tricks Mother Nature gets up to… and there never will be. The riddle of the universe is going to remain just that. The nearest solution to that riddle appeared a couple of centuries ago with a group of scientists in Edinburgh. Those learned fellows assembled weekly to hold discussions on various scientific topics and usually ended the evening with an Ether Party – this involved passing a saucer of ether around and each member sniffing the saucer until he dropped off. On one occasion a member, when he woke up, exclaimed, 'I have found the answer to the riddle of the universe!'

'What is it?' They all cried.

His brow furrowed and after a minute he admitted, 'I don't know: I've forgotten.'

They discussed their disappointment and resolved that next week he should be the only member of the group to sniff ether and that he should try to pay more attention if the answer appeared during his etheric reverie. A week later, surrounded by his eager fellow scientists he alone sniffed ether, became drowsy, slept for a minute or two and then woke with a start.

'Well?' The sober group assembled around him demanded, 'What happened? Did you find the answer?'

'Yes!' He cried from his heart.

'What is it?' The scientists demanded as one.

Briefly his brow furrowed, and then… he slowly recited, 'Higgamus hoggamus, Woman is monogamous… Hoggamus higgamus, Man is polygamous.'

In my view that will do just as well as Big Bangs, black holes or Panspermia, which, resonate less well in my simple mind than the story in Genesis of the Creation and Adam and Eve.

ALTHOUGH I WAS BROUGHT UP WITH CHRISTIAN BELIEFS, to many of which I still adhere, a lifetime of examining various religious doctrines and eyeing the goings-on of the clerics of many sects and religions around the world has led me to question if they know the answer to the mystery of life and existence, or whether there are simply billions of self-deceivers. I call myself an optimistic agnostic, which I guess is more positive than Richard Dawkins' agnostic atheist.

One question which particularly bothers me is that if scientific evidence indicates that mankind, as we know it today, is at least 150 thousand years old, why is it that Christianity is only 2,000 years old and Islam 600 years younger? Did God or Allah have to wait that long before revealing The Truth?

The optimistic part of my personal philosophy will be buoyed by the anticipation that in the final count the plusses of my behaviour through life will outweigh the minuses. So that, assuming there is a pleasant hereafter – with some sort of umpire determining who enters – I can have hope that I will be able to enjoy a slice.

To keep my understanding of the world simple I will accept Mother Nature as she is; I will not waste mental energy pondering where she came from. I hope she will not mind if I continue to degenerate at a comfortably slow rate. I know I'm no good to her anymore, but I do like the world she parents, and yes... all-in-all she is a good mother.

BUT ONE FINAL THOUGHT UPON WHICH TO PONDER – if the universe began with the Big Bang with all matter instantly racing away from the heart of the explosion, the black hole – will it all finish with another Big Bang? This time a huge reversal... with you, your goldfish, your house, the Earth, our solar system and the vast universe rushing to disappear in a flash down a black hole?

And then where do you think you'll be?

12. MY GOD I'M SEVENTY YEARS OLD!

MON DIEU, J'AI SOIXANTE'–DIX ANS!

THREE YEARS AGO, AFTER PRACTISING MEDICINE FOR NEARLY FIVE DECADES, I retired to a little town in Provence. It is great living in glorious countryside among the French in what the local tourist office calls, un climat tonique.

Visiting the doctor:
The other day I visited my doctor to discuss the results of a series of routine tests, I was in good spirits, I'd peeked at them and they were as good as normal, especially for one who likes to indulge year-round in the local delights.

Seventy years young:
'Eh bien,' he said, 'your liver functions are a little aggressif, your blood sugar is still normal but it is rising, and you have gained five kilos since you came here.' Alas, he was right. 'But,' he went on, 'you are only seventy, you are not eighty, you are not old, do something about it, you know what to do.'

Too right, I had been preaching that same message

myself for years and I left his 'cabinet' with those sweet words, you are seventy, you are not old, ringing in my ears. And it's true, these days seventy is not old, it is not the time to sit by the fire with your feet up, it's the time to look to the future, it is the time to develop a my-God-I'm-seventy strategy.

SEVEN STEPS TO KEEP FIT AND HEALTHY IN YOUR SEVENTIES:

Step one:
OBVIOUS – FOLLOW THE DOCTOR'S ADVICE, lose a bit of weight, take some exercise and reduce the, how did he put it? Alimentation excessif.

Step two:
WHEN LOOKING IN THE MIRROR I will not dwell on the hair sprouting out of my ears and nose, the bags under my eyes – and the face gazing back which looks for all the world like my late father's. I will not regard with dismay the brown grave spots appearing on the backs of my hands; the skin that is thinned, the prominent veins and the universal wrinkles. I will positively ignore these trappings of antiquity.

Perhaps like Dracula I should ban all mirrors and, hey, didn't he have a sure recipe for immortality? Alas, not a practical solution. But I have to admit that there are some pretty nifty looking maidens hereabouts and we do have lots of brilliant moonlit nights.

Step three:
KEEP READING AND TAKE ACTION on all the news about life-prolonging things; aspirin reduces the incidence of heart attacks, cancers of the mouth, oesophagus and colon, so take a small daily dose; fibre reduces the risk of colon cancer so start the day with a bowl of high fibre cereal; drink coffee, they say it helps

prevent cirrhosis of the liver (does this mean that I can up the intake of Côtes du Rhône?) and eating an orange or tangerine a day diminishes the risk of lung cancer by thirty per cent.

Whether these pieces of advice are truly ingredients for la vie prolongée needs proper confirmation... but meanwhile there's no harm in taking them. And I gain extra comfort by observing that if I add together all the life-increasing percentages recommended in the course of a week in the tabloid press – by eating more fish and fruit, drinking more red wine and coffee, and so on – by simple arithmetic it is clear that I shall prolong my life by more than a hundred per cent... bonne idée, géniale.

Step four:
KEEP THE BRAIN ACTIVE. A recent study in New York showed that elderly people who stimulated their brains were seventy-five per cent less likely to become demented. Do crosswords, learn a language, develop new hobbies, and above all, socialize.

Step five:
KEEP CHEERFUL. Another recent study has shown that the part of the brain concerned with happiness can stimulate the immune system to work harder. People who are depressed get more colds, colds lead to bronchitis and worse. Part of keeping happy is to have plenty of friends, this means more effort on your part to make new ones and keep old ones. Happiness is also helped along by being of service to others. The father of a friend of mine, at the age of ninety, was regularly delivering meals-on-wheels to youngsters aged seventy ... he died recently, just short of his century.

Step six:
MAKE SURE WHERE YOU LIVE IS AS FALL AND ACCIDENT PROOF as possible. Avoid ladders,

step ladders, loose carpets, ill-fitting footwear, poor illumination, have a fire extinguisher in the kitchen, make sure your locks are secure. Make sure your house is warm in the winter and cool in the summer. Don't smoke, it's never too late to give up. Smoking not only causes cancers, it rots your brain, your heart, your lungs, your arteries, your pancreas, and your gullet... it is also one of the commonest causes of accidental fires.

Step seven:
LIVE IN FRANCE. France has over twenty thousand centenarians and the number is rising year on year.

I HAVE TO ADMIT THAT I HAVE LIVED ANOTHER TEN YEARS SINCE I wrote 'My God I'm Seventy Years Old!' It was originally published on the Internet, without my knowledge. Much to my surprise, some journalist flogged it to a company selling French property who then attached it to their publicity. I received a fee of €20 (£15), that was the first time I had been paid for writing. Over my medical career I had a large number of articles published in medical journals and I had regularly written health columns in the Dubai local dailies during the eighteen years I lived and worked in the Persian Gulf – I still have that wrinkled and grubby €20 note and with it I can join the select association of professional writers in agreeing with Dr Samuel Johnson's aphorism, 'No man but a blockhead ever wrote except for money.'

I treasure that twenty euro note and apart from skeletal degenerative problems in my seventies (hip replacements and back surgery) I have survived and entered my ninth decade with confidence. I shall follow my advice for the seventies; it will be just as valid for the eighties but the additional decade has brought more experience and I can add another five steps in order to:

KEEP GOING IN YOUR EIGHTIES.

Step one:

KEEP LAUGHING: George Bernard Shaw said, 'You don't stop laughing when you grow old; you grow old when you stop laughing.'

Don't turn into a grump – to the old, the world changes only for the worst; standards fall, 'food has no taste these days,' 'the young have no respect,' 'in my day…'etc. If you make a habit of grumbling you'll soon be labelled a miserable old fart, and once you have that reputation, it sticks.

Step two:

DO EXACTLY AS YOU PLEASE, or rather, do exactly as pleases you – 'The years between fifty and seventy are the hardest, you are always being asked to do things and yet you are not yet decrepit enough to turn them down.' T. S. Eliot.

Step three:

LIVE EACH DAY AS IT COMES, don't obsessively think about the future and what it holds. Relish the past, call upon pleasant memories, above all make an effort to enjoy your daily life.

Step four:

MOURN THE LOSS OF OLD FRIENDS and relatives; it's bound to be a recurrent hiccough in your serene senility. But keep the mourning brief, remember the good times with them, and quietly enjoy the minor triumph brought by each of your additional days.

Step five:

IF YOU GET WOBBLY get a stout walking stick. Falling over and banging your head does you no good at all; falls are terminal events, or disastrously handicapping, in thousands of old folks. Exercise – if it doesn't hurt too much – walking helps to keep the leg muscles in trim and lessens the likelihood of falls. If you take medications check with your pharmacist or doctor that they do not cause dizziness.

AND IF YOU STILL HAVE A LIKING FOR ALCOHOL – take extra care in your eighties. Generally octogenarians reduce their intake but, if you are one of those who thinks he can continue to drink like the brave young buck he once was, don't booze it up in the pub around the corner, take a six-pack to bed, it's not so far to fall.

13. HISTORICAL MAMMARIES

QUEEN VICTORIA HAD NINE CHILDREN, ALTHOUGH SHE HATED BABIES – she said they looked like frogs. There were two reasons she had so many. The first was that she and her handsome husband, Prince Albert, were extremely fond of each other and both took delight in bedroom exercise. The second, that she loathed the very thought of breast feeding; all her infants were wet-nursed.

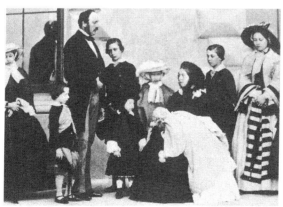

The Queen, the Prince and their children

Lactation is a form of birth control, ovulation is suppressed; but it is not a reliable method, think Irish Catholic families with twenty children. The succession of wet nurses Victoria employed always came from a good class of person, although in 1841 she complained of the drunkenness of the one she had hired to feed the Princess Royal. In Victoria's time there were limited methods of birth control but in 1844, seven years after she ascended the throne, Mr Goodyear, in the United States, vulcanised rubber and rubber condoms became available a decade later. They lacked the sensitivity of later latex models but for the patriotic a picture of Queen Victoria was imprinted on the shaft and for members of the Liberal Party a picture of the Prime Minister, Mr Gladstone. Those early condoms were not popular, they were coarse and one brand had gained the disconcerting reputation of having one dud in every packet. Maybe the happy royal couple knew about these rubber devices but one can be pretty certain they did not use them. Victoria's production line continued until her partner, her beloved Albert, died early, at the age of forty-two.

ALBERT'S PREMATURE DEATH was related to the enthusiastic libido of their first-born son, Edward, later King Edward VII and known as 'Bertie' in the family. He had a liking for the ladies – a taste he cultivated, honed and turned into a life-long pursuit. Early in that career, when he was a student at Cambridge University, gossip in gentlemen's clubs in London and the foreign press held that he had 'placed young Nellie Clifden [an actress] in a very delicate situation.' In fact Bertie had entered adult life in Ireland while on temporary duty with the army – fellow officers decided to help Bertie to mature and smuggled Nellie, a willing teacher, into his tent one night.

Prince Albert was furious when news of the scandal reached his ears; although he and his wife were dedicated to cavorting between the sheets, that was their business, and, unusually for royalty of those times – or maybe, of any time – they maintained a devoted and strictly monogamous relationship.

Albert went to Cambridge to sort out his wayward son. It was just before Christmas 1861, it was bitterly cold and he travelled by coach to and from Windsor Castle. We don't know how, or even if, he sorted out Bertie, but Prince Albert became ill on the return journey and when he arrived back at Windsor took immediately to his bed. A committee of royal physicians was summoned and diagnosed a severe chill… within days the chill led to a fever which was said to have assumed a typhoid character. Twelve days after his return Albert was dead. No more progeny, no need for wet nurses, and Victoria wore black until she died forty years later.

WET NURSING HAS A LONG HISTORY. The Bible gives an account of how Pharaoh's daughter, Bitya, while she was having a dip in the Nile, found a three month old baby boy in a papyrus cradle among the bulrushes. At that time her father, fearing the Israelis were becoming too uppity, was killing off male Hebrew babies by having his soldiers throw them in the river – a story repeated by King Herod at Christmas fourteen centuries later.

When Bitya first saw the baby it cried, melting her heart. She was so touched that she plucked him from the cradle, immediately spotting that the baby was a 'he' and was Hebrew, she did not hand him to her father's soldiers, she ordered a girl she found lurking nearby, 'Find a Hebrew wet nurse for this baby and tell her that I will pay her wages to suckle him.'

She called the baby Moses, which means, the plucked one. It so happened that the girl she spoke to was Miriam, the baby's sister, who had been hanging around waiting to see what would happen to her little baby brother. Not surprisingly she was instantly able to come up with a wet nurse, a woman called Jochebed – Moses' mother – Moses was wet nursed by his mother.

Wet nursing by animals has a long history but most stories are made of the stuff of legend and many have remarkably similar storylines. Perhaps the earliest recorded was in the writings of the Father of History, Herodotus, who wrote of Cyrus the King of Persia (600-530BC) that he was suckled by a bitch. The grandfather of Cyrus was told that his grandson would depose him. The news came through unpleasant dreams his daughter experienced towards the end of her pregnancy. Not long after birth Cyrus was handed to a servant with orders to get rid of him. Reluctant to murder the baby, the servant left Cyrus on a hillside.

A wandering (and fortuitously lactating) wild dog found Cyrus and suckled him until he was discovered by a shepherd. The shepherd took him home and he and his wife cared for Cyrus until he became a man. An alternative story is that the servant gave Cyrus to a huntsman telling him to kill the baby. It so happened that the huntsman's wife had just delivered a stillborn child and so could suckle Cyrus – her name was Spako – which translates as, dog.

A similar story with Paris, son of Priam, King of Troy, towards the end of her pregnancy Paris's mother dreamed that she had given birth to a flaming torch. A seer declared that this foretold the downfall of Troy and the head priestess at the temple of Apollo confirmed the warning. Priam gave the newborn Paris to his chief herdsman with instructions to kill him but the herdsman could not bring himself to do the deed and left Paris on the side of Mount Ida. A passing (again fortuitously lactating) she-bear came upon Paris and suckled him until his rearing was taken over by a shepherd. Paris had a distinguished life; he eloped with Helen, Queen of Sparta, and shot an arrow into the heel of Achilles.

Telephus was yet another whose infancy was marred by his Grandfather, King Aleus of Tegea. He had been told by the Oracle that he would be overthrown by his grandson. Grandfather hit on the idea of consigning his daughter, Auge, to the Temple of Athena as a virginal priestess. He felt sure that the obligatory vow of chastity would put an end to the prophecy. Nevertheless, she willingly submitted to a visitor to the temple, the irresistible demi-god Hercules; later claiming that she had been violated. She called the baby Telephus. Worried that the infant's cries could be heard in the temple, and fearing discovery and retribution, she had Telephus abandoned on the side of Mount Parthenon. Somehow his father, Hercules, got to know and directed help to him, in the form of a lactating doe.

Thereafter the story becomes complicated and there are variations. Having survived infancy, Telephus was, by some accounts, brought up by, the customary shepherd family and as a young man journeyed to Tegea. He was adopted by King Teuthras when he was young and subsequently became a heroic and famous general. As a reward for winning a battle for him King Teuthras gave Telephus a beautiful woman, an ex-priestess he had adopted called Auge. Auge was given in betrothal to Telephus, who did not know she was his mother. But the flame of passion for Hercules still burned in Auge's breast and on the wedding night she took a knife to bed to kill Telephus. Fortunately the semi-divine Hercules again spotted what was going on and shot a bolt of lightning which thrust the two apart – they instantly recognised each other for what they were, mother and son.

According to legend the founder of Rome, Romulus, and his twin Remus, were also born of a temple virgin sworn to chastity. She was called Rhea Silvia and was ordered to the temple, not by her father the king, Numitor, but by his brother, Amulius, who had seized power and murdered all the other male heirs. Rhea Silvia claimed to have been inseminated by the god Mars, or maybe it was Hercules, she wasn't too sure.

Uncle Amulius had the twins abandoned in the river Tiber, but miraculously they survived. They were found and wet nursed by a she wolf. They were later weaned by the introduction of solids brought by a woodpecker. The traditional shepherd and his wife reared them to adulthood. They became brilliant soldiers and won victories galore. They decided to build a magnificent city but bitterly disagreed on where to build it. They fought each other and Romulus killed Remus. Had Remus won, the capital of Italy would have been called Reme and be inhabited by Remans.

In the heyday of Rome, female slaves who were lactating were sought after and fetched a high price. A road in Rome, the Via Lattaria, was lined every morning by milk-laden young women. Roman businessmen on their way to the office could put down their brief cases and have a milky breakfast for a few copper coins, and for another copper or two carry away a clay bottle full of breast milk for their elevenses.

Wealthy Roman ladies had no objection to their husbands impregnating their slave girls and themselves at about the same time. The slave girl could then suckle both babies, allowing the Roman lady to keep her figure and resume her social life.

IN THE EIGHTEENTH AND NINETEENTH CENTURIES animals wet nursing children was practised in foundling hospitals. Lactating donkeys or goats provided several daily feeds; the infants would be held to the teat by nursemaids sitting on stools. Alternatively the infants were laid in stable stalls and at set times the donkeys would be led in and straddle the infants who would take a teat. Not infrequently a donkey would bond with and suckle one particular child.

Animal wet nurses were used therapeutically in treating babies with congenital syphilis, which was common and easy to recognise at birth. Treatment for syphilis at the time was with mercury compounds which were introduced into the feed of the goats which were suckling the infants. The mercury compounds were absorbed and secreted in the goat's milk, and thus delivered to the syphilitic suckling. Alas, the results were poor; no improvement in the infants, the goats went as mad as hatters – or maybe as giddy as goats – and died of mercury poisoning.

Carl Linnaeus (1707-1778), the botanist, expressed concern that infants suckled by animals might take on the animal characteristics of the wet nurse. He went as far as to suggest that for a child to acquire great strength and courage a lioness should be employed, there is no account of this actually happening.

You would think that humans suckling animals would not be countenanced but it was recommended as therapy for hardening over-delicate nipples and there was a vogue for using it to treat of infection of the womb after delivery. It was known empirically that nipple stimulation led to uterine contraction. Now we know that nipple stimulation leads to the release from the pituitary gland of a hormone, oxytocin, which is made in the hypothalamus. Oxytocin has many actions which include the first letting down of the secretion of breast milk and at the same time causing uterine contractions. To this day, if there is delay in the third stage of labour (delivery of the placenta, the after-birth), midwives put the child to the mother's breast to cause contractions of the uterus to encourage expulsion of the placenta.

Mary Wollstonecraft had puerperal fever and died ten days after the delivery of her second daughter, Mary, who was to marry the poet Shelley and write Frankenstein. She was given puppies to suckle in the belief that doing so would cause contraction of the uterus and expel the infected material within. Although the theory has merit, in practice little benefit accrued. Puerperal sepsis is not confined to the uterus; doomed new mothers die of generalised septicaemia leading to multi-organ failure.

In the eighteenth century wet nursing in France became an organised industry. Recommanderesses, the equivalent of brothel madams, and also known as Pimps of Suckling, set up offices in Paris. Twenty-one thousand babies were born in the capital each year but comparatively few were fed by their natural mother or a wet nurse, une nourrice, who lived in the family home.

With thousands of babies to be fed every day it became necessary for the infants to go to the wet nurses and a system of transportation was set up. Cartloads of suckling infants were collected in the early morning and sent to women in the banlieue, the suburbs, encompassing Paris. The carts were rickety and jolted, bumped and juddered their way through the capital's potholed streets. Unfortunate infants might be tossed out of the cart or fall through holes in the floor and be crushed under the cart's wheels. Of the suckling infants not transported in wagons, most were stuffed into large wicker baskets and carried on the backs of men, again with a high mortality rate – if they didn't freeze to death in winter they suffocated in summer.

BABIES WERE DELIVERED DAILY TO WET NURSES, who were usually sluts rearing several at the same time. A number of infants stayed permanently with wet nurses until they achieved weaning, providing they survived that long. Many nourrices lived in hovels with open fires and animals snuffling around. There were stories of some infants being eaten by pigs and of others dying a horrible death if a spark ignited the cradle. Those who lapsed into coma through malnutrition or illness would be taken to a nearby fountain, whose icy waters had healing properties, and dunked; that resuscitated a few but more often polished them off.

In 1769 King Louis XV (The Well-Beloved) declared that the industry should be regulated. Henceforth carts carrying babies should have enough planks on the floor to stop them falling through and cart tops should have hoops covered in canvas to prevent them popping over the side.

Despite the appalling mortality rate in suckling infants – estimated at ninety per cent at the end of the Ancien Régime, the French Revolution – the practice continued. Many deaths went unreported to the parents and les nourrices continued to pocket money for suckling infants already interred.

For the richer classes, la petite bourgeoisie, artisans, and small businesses, les nourrices provided a vital service. Like their Roman forebears the rich and middle classes used wet nurses widely, not only to preserve their own figures and beauty but to be able to be sexually active… It was widely believed that the Bible forbade sexual relations with a woman who was breast feeding.

From the end of nineteenth century there was a reaction to the deplorable industry of les nourrices. It was no longer believed that giving the milk of an animal, goat, sheep or cow, would convey the bestial qualities of that animal to the infant or that a foreign wet nurse would convey her temperament, character and morals through her milk, even black wet nurses became acceptable.

Doctors tried to convince mothers that breast feeding could not make them ugly; they also scared them by telling them that there was danger for women who abandoned breast feeding early. That, for instance, the lactating woman's own milk would seep back into her body causing lunacy and even more serious to the young Parisian mother, unexpelled milk would lead to seriously drooping breasts.

Popular opinion demanded strict regulation of the activities of les nourrices. The organisation was taken out of the hands of the Pimps of Suckling and a Bureau of Wet Nurses was set up. Pay was regulated and wet nurses could be selected in the knowledge that each had been approved by a doctor who had examined la nourrice; seized and squeezed her nipples, tasted her milk, evaluated its quality and issued a signed certificate: 'testé et approuvé'

– tested and approved. A priest was also involved to provide a certificate of good morality.

With proper regulation the industry gained respect and wet nurses, far from being slovens, assumed the premier place in the hierarchy of domestics in the houses of the Paris rich. She was paid well (110 francs a month); had her own quarters, her own coachman, and fed well in order to make sure that she would give the infant the best quality milk. To make sure that she was fed well the choicest piece of meat on the dinner table was reserved for her and became known as, 'le morceau de la nourrice,' – the wet-nurse's piece. The careers of wet-nurses usually didn't last much more than a decade but in that time they were able to save enough to build and retire to pretty houses – which naturally became known as 'maisons du lait,' – Houses of Milk.

Wet-nursing in France did not wane until World War I when safe, easy, and inexpensive artificial infant feeding became available. Wet nursing in France had practically disappeared by the nineteen twenties.

And what of wet nursing on the other side of that stretch of water the French call La Manche, the sleeve, and deride the Anglo-Saxons for calling it the English Channel? Never an industry, nor much of a cultural phenomenon, wet nursing was most widely practised among the rich. In 1863 the weekly Medical Times and Gazette counselled that, 'In cases where it is inadvisable to give the child to the breast, amongst the higher classes, who can afford to have a wet nurse, a good one should be procured at once. Amongst the lower orders the child should be fed in great part upon the bottle.'

If, however, one subscribed to the generally held belief that the lower and labouring classes were unclean and immoral and would transmit these traits, how could one obtain a reliable wet nurse of quality? The answer was to apply to a Lying-In (Maternity) Hospital. Queen Charlotte's, the biggest lying-in hospital in London, advertised that, 'Wet nurses can always be supplied on application to the Matron.' It was unlikely that a trollop could pass the eagle-eyed inspection of the Charlotte's matron.

IN ENGLAND THERE WERE IRREGULARITIES and situations which paralleled the worst aspects of the French system. In the middle of the nineteenth century the registrar of the London district of Marylebone recorded nineteen deaths in children less than a year old in the month of August. He recorded that most of them had been, 'brought up by hand and were illegitimate.'

Money was tight in those days; some girls viewed wet nursing as a good alternative to poorly paid drudgery. But in order to produce milk they had to get pregnant and when their baby was delivered it would be given to a relative or friend for hand rearing. While the wet nurse was paid to suckle to some middle class whelp her own infant was fed an inadequate and unsuitable diet; commonly these infants did not survive beyond the age of four or five months.

Burial Clubs provided a final pay-off for wet nurses. In poverty stricken families an infant's death would carry even more tragedy if the family was so poor it could not afford a proper funeral. To the family's everlasting shame the tiny corpse would be consigned in a simple shroud to a communal pauper's grave.

Churches, trades unions and charitable groups formed what were called Friendly Societies which promoted Burial Clubs and for a small weekly sum provided payment of funeral and interment expenses. There were a number of these societies and an unscrupulous wet nurse who had charge of a sickly infant which was likely to die would enrol it in several Burial Clubs; the record was nineteen.

When I was a medical student in London, over half a century ago, I was taught that compared with bottle-feeding, breast-feeding was much better. There were several reasons: the milk came in handy, attractive containers, it was always at the right temperature, was instantly available, cheap, and didn't need sterilizing. Moreover it contained protective substances, such as immunoglobulins, which coat the baby's intestine, like a lick of paint, and prevented infections.

But as I remember, one crucially important advantage was not stressed at that time, maternal-child bonding... which, incidentally, also occurs in children habitually bottle fed by their own mothers.

An example of the effects of a lack of bonding between mother and son was told in the legend of Oedipus. The parents of Oedipus consulted the Oracle at Delphi because of their childlessness. The Oracle told them that if they had a son he would be destined to kill his father, Laius, and marry his mother, Jocasta.

Inevitably Jocasta bore Laius a son. For some mysterious reason, but vital to the story, Laius tied the infant's ankles tightly together and then told Jocasta to kill him. She found herself unable to do that, so she abandoned him in the wilderness. Fortunately he was found by a wandering shepherd who called him Oedipus – an interesting name, it literally means swollen foot. Doctors describe the fluid in swellings due to fluid accumulation as 'oedema.'

As would be expected in a mythological story, the Oracle's prophecy came true. Oedipus met his father on a narrow road, they were in their chariots and neither would give way. In possibly the world's first account of Road Rage they quarrelled ferociously, fought, and Oedipus killed his father. Later Oedipus met Jocasta, didn't know she was his mother, fell in love with her and they married.

SIGMUND FREUD WAS SUCKLED BY A WET NURSE. His mother, Amalia, was the second, or possibly third, wife of Jacob, his father. She was quite a dish and twenty years younger than Jacob. As a small boy he watched her undress in a sleeper on a train and experienced a penile awakening. That possibly wouldn't have happened if Amalia had breast fed him.

In 1921 a Finnish anthropologist called Westermarck came up with the theory that early bonding, parental or sibling, desensitises sexual attraction later in life. Normally brothers and sisters find no sexual attraction in post-pubertal life; but if they are separated at a very early age and meet for the first time as young adults they may fall violently in love.

Maybe Sophocles, who wrote his play and called it Oedipus Rex, already knew the substance of the theory Westermarck would enunciate over two millennia later. Sigmund Freud didn't, he came to ascribe many human psychological frailties to sexually orientated causes and popularised his Oedipus Complex – contemporary psychologists express doubts concerning his theories and it is likely that some of his concepts had their origin in personal experiences. Perhaps he, subconsciously, transformed his own early sexual awakening when he described what he called the 'phallic phase of sexual development' which he said occurred between the ages of three and six. Just think, if Amalia Freud had breast fed little Sigi we would not have the Oedipus Complex and so-called Freudian Slips would have to find another name.

Throughout history women's breasts have been a source of admiration. There is on record a certain lady in ancient Greece who had a pair which the world has not seen the like of since.

She was nicknamed Phryne, which translates from the Greek as toad. Unlikely as it sounds it is said that the nickname referred to the colour of the skin of her face, a sallow, toad-like tone which was regarded as highly attractive in those days. She was not only extremely attractive, she was witty and clever. She put her natural endowments to such good use that in no time she became very rich, so rich that she offered to rebuild the walls of

Thebes on condition that the words *destroyed by Alexander, restored by Phryne, the courtesan,* were inscribed. Such presumptuousness irritated the elders who declined her offer, and who, because she also made many rash utterances about Greek deities, tried to nail her by charging her with blasphemy.

Phryne was defended by the great orator Hyperides, who, when it looked as though the verdict was going against her, leaned forward, seized her dress, tore it and displayed her bosoms to the jury – the jury (all male, I suspect) gasped and instantly acquitted her.

But if the question is asked: Whose breasts are best? The answer has to be the biological mother's... provided that she didn't use a wet nurse.

14. PROVENCE – THE DIVINE CHOICE

> I breathe in and draw toward me the air
> that I feel coming from Provence;
> everything that comes from there pleases me,
> such that when I hear good told of it
> I listen with a smile.

> Peire Vidal, troubadour (1175-1205)

IN THE SECOND CENTURY BEFORE CHRIST ROME DEFEATED THE LIGURIANS who, together with immigrant Celts, occupied the Northwest Mediterranean coast from the mouth of the river Ebro in present-day Spain to the river Arno in Italy. The Romans established their headquarters in Aix-en-Provence and military colonies in Massilia (later called Marseille), Arles and Narbonne. The countryside so delighted Caesar with its charm, fertility, and beauty that he decided it should be an integral part of Rome. He called the region Romana Provincia, a name which was later shortened to Provence.

Provence has attracted man since time immemorial; relics of tools dating back a million years and human settlements, six hundred thousand years old, have been uncovered along the Mediterranean coast of Provence. The coastal area, known to the world as the Côte d'Azur, and called by the English, The French Riviera, stretches from St Tropez to the Italian border. Much of the land of the littoral is arid and desolate with bare rocks rising out of patches of green; but it has a pleasing climate, attractive beaches, clear blue seas and welcoming natural harbours. Numbers of visitors increased rapidly with the coming of the railways and the fashionable English discovering it in late Victorian and Edwardian times.

After the Second World War the French Riviera became once again the playground of the ultra-wealthy. Speculators had a field day and the world's rich colonised the Riviera beneath its brilliant-blue skies and a coast lapped by seas reflecting the deep azure, cloudless skies above. Super-rich socialites, media celebrities, Arab billionaires, and Russian oligarchs gamble away vast sums in casinos while their hugely expensive yachts cram the berths of the harbours of Nice and Cannes.

The awe-inspiring beauty of the landscape of the interior of Provence stretches from the snow-capped mountains of the Southern Alps to the flat plains and marshes of the Camargue. Provence, away from the showy, meretricious French Riviera, attracts the world; it is intriguing, unique, and beautiful. Its sunshine is almost guaranteed, and the rich Provençal foods with fine local wines, combine to excite the palate. Add to them the heady perfume of its vegetation, the maquis; the magnificently preserved Roman buildings; amphitheatres in Arles and Orange, the enormous aqueduct of the Pont du Gard, the vestiges in Vaison la Romaine and one's spinning mind is easily transported to the glories of Rome. The Papal Palace in Avignon speaks of the time when Provence was the centre of the Christian world. The charming and delightful villages perchés on the summits of hills and on mountainsides speak of yet another historical epoch. Perched villages are scattered all over Provence and recall the dreadful events of the thirteenth and fourteenth centuries. In that era France was pillaged, its crops destroyed, and populations slaughtered by bands of mounted soldiers, mostly English, called Chevauchées. Being perched on a hilltop was then a matter of survival and the view was admired, not for its beauty, but for the ability to spot marauders from afar.

It is easy to imagine that Provence was specially fashioned by the hand of Divine Providence... perhaps in the beginning by the pantheon of the Gods of Rome and later honed from the Christian headquarters in Avignon. That Hand is still at work, the French take enormous pride in Provence and the preservation of its culture and history.

By that same divine hand a group of the earliest Christians were directed to the shores of Provence. According to legend, in the middle of the first century Anno Domini, a boatload of early Christian Jews disembarked on a beach about two hundred kilometres to the west of the Riviera, they were fleeing persecution by non-Christian Jews in their homeland. The boat, a miracle in itself, was rudderless, had no sails and no provisions, but guided by the Divine Hand it traversed the Mediterranean Sea and even stopped to pick up another passenger in Egypt. The boat made land on the shore of the Camargue, the part of Provence which is formed by the delta of the river Rhône. The settlement founded where those persecuted Christians landed became the capital of the Camargue and was called Les Saintes Maries de la Mer (The Sainted Marys of the Sea). After disembarkation, two of the oldest of the Marys stayed behind, converted the locals and lived out their lives there. All the other passengers left Les Saintes Maries de la Mer and spread the Gospel of Christ across Europe.

The Divine Hand further blessed Provence by bathing it in a light of intense clarity. The extraordinary quality of the light is attributed by the more sanguine to the proximity of the Alps and the cleansing effect of the powerful wind of Provence, the Mistral. No matter what the true cause, the light and scenery attracted artists such as Renoir, Matisse, Van Gogh, Picasso, and Chagall. The native Provençal artist Cézanne, born near Aix, was drawn back to his roots after studying in Paris. After he returned he repeatedly painted nearby Mont Saint-Victoire, no less than sixty times. Cézanne was enthralled by the way the magical properties of the Provençal light wrought an ever-changing vista of the mountain.

The Giant of Provence, its tallest mountain – Mont Ventoux – was another blessing. It provided sanctuary for the Maquis, the French Resistance of World War II. Its forests and scrubland provided shelter for the young men who fought the Nazi German army, the Werhmacht, which was supported by a more cruel foe – fellow French countrymen, collaborators armed by the Nazis – the infamous Milice Française (more of which later).

THE GREAT WIND OF PROVENCE, THE MISTRAL, derives its name from the old Provençal word for *masterly*. The Mistral is created when there is an anticyclone in the Bay of Biscay and an area of low pressure in the Gulf of Genoa. The wind accelerates as it blows down the valley of the Rhône and does not completely expend its energy until it crosses the sea to reach North Africa. While other parts of France are having clouds and storms, the Mistral cleanses the air of Provence; blowing away clouds, humidity, dust and pollution, and leaving a bright, deep-blue, sun-drenched sky.

The Mistral is most prevalent in the winter and spring and, although less frequent, it is more than welcome in the summer as it provides relief after days of scorching heat and rising humidity – the air the day after a summer Mistral is unbelievably sweet-smelling, fresh and cool. The Mistral blows in multiples of three days, up to twelve. It has such a malignant potential for turning minds that in the past if a man murdered his wife, after days and nights of continuously screeching wind, magistrates would not regard him as culpable – whether the wife would be similarly exculpated is not mentioned in local lore. The artist, van Gogh, a man with a fragile personality at the best of times, was said to have been afflicted by the Mistral which together with absinthe could produce a mixture of lethal potential and might account for much of his erratic behaviour.

The river Rhône is the aorta, the main artery of Provence, and is to Provence what great rivers like the Nile, the Yangtze, the Thames, and the Euphrates are to the lands they traverse. Since pre-history the Rhône has enabled commerce, industry and travel. It rises in Switzerland and keeps Lake Geneva topped up before it proceeds on its way to France. Before the days of railroads and highways the great river made it possible for cities along its banks, from Lyon to Avignon, to trade by boat with the Mediterranean port of Marseille.

THE ROMANS ESTABLISHED VINEYARDS in the valley of the Rhône but in the fifth century, with the collapse of the Roman Empire, interest in wine production waned. Happily it was resuscitated by wine-loving popes when the Papacy moved from Rome to Avignon at the beginning of the fourteenth century.

Buy why choose Avignon? In 1305, after the death of Pope Benedict XI and a year-long dispute between French and Italian cardinals, the king of France, Philip IV, engineered the election of the Archbishop of Bordeaux as the new Pope. The new pope took the name Clement V. Like all his papal successors in Avignon he was French and on good terms with his monarch. Pope Clement refused to go to Rome because he was in mortal fear of the ongoing strife affecting the senior hierarchy of the Church there. He first established his court at Carpentras, capital of the Comtat de Venaissin, already a pontifical state. Later he moved a few miles to the west, to Avignon; the reason for that move is unclear. Although owned by the Papacy, Avignon had a reputation for being one of the grubbiest and most dissolute cities in Christendom.

CLEMENT V DIED IN 1314 AND WAS SUCCEEDED BY POPE JOHN XXII in 1316. Again there was an interregnum because the electors, the cardinals, could not agree on a choice. And again it was a French king, Philip V, who in 1316 organised a conclave of twenty three cardinals in Lyon, and directed them to appoint as Pope the Cardinal-Bishop of Porto (who had been appointed to that post by Pope Clement V). He took the name of Pope John XXII.

Pope John XXII was the pope responsible for regenerating interest in viticulture in the south of the Rhône valley. The wines became known generally as *Vins du Pape* – wines of the Pope, and when he constructed a castle on the north bank of the Rhône, a few kilometres from Avignon, the appellation of the wines of the immediate surrounding area became *'Chateauneuf du Pape'* (New Castle of the Pope). Pope John XXII was, however, not responsible for today's exorbitant prices of Chateauneuf du Pape wines. That happened seven centuries later when an American wine critic extolled the virtues of the Chateauneuf du Pape wines. Until then they had been regarded as rustic and holding little appeal to the wine connoisseur. Now there are plenty of wines of the southern Rhone valley with the appellation of Côtes du Rhône Villages AOC which are of at least equal quality, yet they do not have the cachet, or the price, of the wines of the area of the Pope's New Castle.

In early 1317, while journeying back to Avignon from Lyon, where he had been enthroned, Pope John XXII was feeling unwell. So unwell that he ordered his driver to stop the coach so that he could take a rest. He demanded a drink and was brought a glass of the local wine. Within a minute he exclaimed something like, 'God's blood! That did me a power of good… Bring me another!'

After downing the second glass he felt well enough to continue on his way. But first he asked, 'Where are we? What is this place?'

On being told, 'It is the town of Valréas, Your Holiness,' he commanded:

'Buy it, and buy all the vineyards around it.'

The area was in the Drôme, just outside the border of the Department of Vaucluse in northern Provence, and to this day is known as l'Enclave des Papes (the Papal Enclave). One can but reflect that there is only one 'illness' which is so readily relieved by a couple of generous glasses of wine… a hangover.

PETRARCH (1304-1374), SCHOLAR, POET, HUMANIST and one of the authors of the Literary Renaissance was highly critical of the Papal Court in Avignon. In his youth his family had moved to live near the city and he had spent the years of his early adult life there, at the court of Pope Clement V. Petrarch called Avignon, 'The Babylon of the West.' He scorned the rich papal trappings and the corruption of the court. He had studied law at Montpellier and Bologna but became disenchanted with the mercenary nature of lawyers and embarked on a career in the Church – but that was another career he was destined not to follow.

Petrarch recorded with precision that he abandoned his religious vocation at eleven o'clock on the morning of 26 April 1327 while attending morning service at the church of St Claire in Avignon. There, he announced, he had seen the beauty who was to become the queen of his heart, Laura. She was beautiful, fair, dignified, slender, modest, and seventeen years old but, unfortunately for Petrarch, she was married. Her husband was Hugues de Sade – an ancestor of the notorious Marquis – and she rejected Petrarch. It is possible that Laura never again gave him a thought. For Petrarch, however, Laura became an obsession, a figment of his imagination which he beautified and idolised all his days.

Following Laura's rejection Petrarch retreated to Fontaine-de-Vaucluse, a small town to the east of Avignon, the mysterious source of the river Sorgue. There he took a house; listened to the waters, brooded, and wrote sonnets to his beloved Laura. Evidently there were diversions to take his mind off brooding because there he fathered a daughter in 1343, she was called Francesca. A generation later, in 1377, he had a son, Giovanni, in Avignon, but there are no references to a Mrs Petrarch.

PRECISELY TWENTY-ONE YEARS AFTER PETRARCH had first spotted her, Laura died, on the very same date, 26 April (1348), and at the very hour that he had first seen her at the church of St Claire in Avignon. She may have died of the Black Death – rampant that year, or pulmonary tuberculosis. She had given birth to eleven children and as Petrarch had not seen her for so many years one supposes that although he still carried in his mind his original vision of her loveliness she had undoubtedly changed in appearance – to the maternal figure of a woman aged by multiple pregnancies and twenty-one years.

In April 1326, while living at Fontaine-de-Vaucluse, Petrarch climbed Mont Ventoux with his brother and two servants. It was a tough, steep climb; no roads, no paths, treacherous and dense undergrowth. At the summit he marvelled at the majestic views, ruminated for hours and discovered his inner-self. This affected his outlook on life and his writings. He eventually returned to his native Italy where he died at the age of seventy, another victim of the Black Death.

Four centuries later another Provençal character, destined to become one of France's greatest writers and a poet laureate in literature, was born near Avignon, in the Bouches du Rhône. He was Frédéric Mistral and he had the good fortune to be born to a wealthy family, so that throughout his life he was able to concentrate on his literary works. He loved his native Provence and formed a movement to revive and preserve the Provençal language, a dialect of Occitan. Mistral said of Provence:

'QUAND LE BON DIEU EN VIENT A DOUTER DU MONDE, IL SE RAPPEL QU'IL A CREE   LA PROVENCE.'

'When the Good Lord had any doubts about the world [he had made] he reminded himself that he had created Provence.'

15. SAINTLY GOINGS-ON IN PROVENCE

OVER A DECADE AGO I RETIRED TO LIVE IN FRANCE, in a small market town, at the foot of Mont Ventoux. In many years this mountain, known as le Géant de Provence, provides one of the major challenges of international cycle racing, a mountain stage in the Tour de France.

On one unlucky Friday the thirteenth, in July 1967, on the thirteenth stage of the Tour de France, it proved a mortal challenge for the British world champion cyclist, Tom Simpson. In the blazing sun the massed group of cyclists climbed the steep, tortuous twenty-one kilometres from the base to the top. Tom was close to the front but as the summit drew near he wobbled and fell off. Helpers rushed to him and as he was picked up they heard him hoarsely implore, 'Put me back on my bike.'

Those were his last words. He was taken by police helicopter to hospital in Avignon but died later that day without regaining consciousness. An autopsy revealed high blood levels of amphetamine. Amphetamine tablets were found in the pockets of his shorts and a large supply was found in his hotel room. He had also swallowed a quantity of brandy to ease his saddle soreness. In 1967 performance-enhancing drugs were not banned substances.

The French had long adored Tom; they took him to their hearts and called him, 'Mr Tom.' Close to the top of Mont Ventoux a granite memorial with an inscribed polished plaque was erected to him at the roadside where he fell. To this day cyclists who climb the mountain leave tributes on the memorial plinth, bunches of flowers, messages and drink bottles. To mark the thirtieth anniversary of his death his daughters, Joanne and Jane, added a plaque inscribed, 'No mountain too high.'

If canonization was by popular acclaim there is no doubt that the memorial would have been dedicated to 'Saint Tom Simpson,' although perhaps his motto, "If ten will kill you, take nine and win," would not have featured in the Vatican's Saints' Roll.

Had Tom become one of Provence's saints he would be the only one with irrefutable evidence of mortal existence; all the others are the stuff of legend. With non-existent contemporary records the stories of the Christian saints were handed down through the generations by word of mouth. Written religious records do exist but their authenticity is doubtful as they were written so many centuries after the miraculous events they relate. Naturally all have a Christian theme and were accepted with the unquestioning faith of the day.

At that time, centuries before the dawn of the Age of Enlightenment, everybody; rich or poor, noble or base, had religion for moral sustenance. For particular troubles, special saints to whom they could appeal for help – certainly more effective than doing nothing – and, so what if cynics invoke a saintly placebo effect? In those harsh times all they had for their physical welfare were intercessory prayers and herbal remedies… what today one would call, complementary or alternative therapies.

Throughout the Christian world the stories of saintly goings-on are rich, interesting, and full of whimsy; none more so than the tales of the Saints of Provence.

THERE ARE THOUSANDS OF SAINTS in France, several allocated to each day of the year. For example, there are three for 29 February. First, St Albinus, in the sixth century he gained grace by ransoming slaves. Second, St Bridget, strictly speaking Irish but available in France; she is the Bridget who spoke to St Patrick and persuaded him to declare that yearning maidens could propose marriage on Leap Year's Day. Third was the tenth century St Oswald, he was English but spent his middle years as a monk in France – famously St Oswald disciplined disorderly clerics while washing a dozen pairs of feet every day.

On the north side of Mont Ventoux at seven hundred metres above the pretty medieval village of Beaumont du Ventoux, stands a simple chapel built in 1684 and dedicated to St Sidoine. Sidoine (or Sidonius, or Sidon, or Cedonius) was the man in the Bible, blind from birth, whose sight was immediately restored when Jesus mixed his own saliva with soil to form a paste which he then applied to Sidoine's eyelids – but how did he end up in France?

We will come to that after mentioning that there had been a chapel previously on that very same site dedicated to another saint, St Elzéar (1285-1323). St Elzéar was of noble birth and ostentatiously religious from the very beginning of his life, the infant Elzéar refused milk from his wet nurse on Fridays and on days of fasting. He married Delphine of Glandèves (1284-1358), also of noble stock. On their wedding night Elzéar's bride announced that she had taken a vow of life-long virginity. Instead of throwing himself, or even Delphine, off the nearest parapet, Elzéar immediately made his own vow of permanent celibacy.

The couple lived lives of great piety; competing with each other in prayer, self-flagellation, mortification of the flesh, and charitable works. So pure and devoted were their lives that both Elzéar and Delphine were canonized at the same time by Pope Urban V – who as it happened was their godson. Pope Gregory XI completed the simultaneous husband-and-wife elevation to sainthood in 1371.

ST SIDOINE CAME TO FRANCE AS ONE OF A BOATLOAD OF EARLY CHRISTIAN JEWS fleeing the Holy Land and persecution by traditional Jews. The actual date is unclear but it was probably between 41 and 46AD. Times had become decidedly uncomfortable for Christian converts. The Jews had recently stoned to death St Stephen who had accused them of murdering Jesus. At about the same time King Herod Agrippa (continuing the family tradition started by his grandfather, King Herod the Great, of chopping off people's heads) had St James the Greater beheaded for preaching the Gospel. The Nazarenes, as the early Christians were known, were in fear of their lives and decided to flee Palestine.

They were led to a beach north of Caesarea by none other than Paul, originally called Saul, who was one of the most enthusiastic tormentors of Christians until he converted to their faith on the road to Damascus. He subsequently became St Paul the Apostle to the Gentiles. Paul took the Nazarenes to a boat on the beach. There are many legends about the journey of this boat, and its passengers from the East to the West of the Mediterranean.

How many boarded the boat is disputed. One legend mentions seventeen, which included two children... one of whom was called Sara and was alleged to be the daughter of Jesus and Mary Magdalene. According to another account there were seventy-two disciples. The boat was a miracle in itself. It had no sails; no oars, no rudder and no provisions; but all hazards were overcome thanks to the hand of Divine Providence guiding it.

As it happened a parallel legend occurred at about the same time; it concerned St James the Greater, whose martyrdom had made up the minds of the Nazarenes to flee Palestine. The body and head of the martyr were placed in a stone coffin and carried by angels and favourable winds through the Pillars of Hercules (the Straits of Gibraltar) to land at Finisterre in Spain. He was taken inland and buried in his stone coffin in an unmarked grave in the middle of a field.

St James's tomb was discovered eight centuries later when a hermit heard music and saw a brilliant light hovering over a particular spot in the middle of a field. The King of Spain declared the tomb to be that of St Iago (Iago, Spanish for James) and a church was built over it. The Pope sanctified the area and miracles ensued, the most important being St Iago's part in finally ridding Spain of the invading Moors in 1492. Enlarged into a cathedral it became one of Christianity's great pilgrimage shrines, St Iago de Compostella. Pilgrims are promised forgiveness of their sins, particularly when they make the pilgrimage in a year when the Feast Day of St Iago (25 July) falls on a Sunday.

To return to the shipload bound for Provence. In some texts the remains of the corpse of St Anne, the mother of the Virgin Mary, are included in the bill of lading. She had been dead for fifty years and those early Christians feared that her tomb and body would be profaned by non-Christian Jews. Her relics were eventually taken by one of the passengers, St Lazarus, to her final resting place in Apt, near Avignon. The church built to house her tomb collapsed in disrepair after five centuries and the mortal remains of St Anne were lost forever... apparently.

The ruins of the church were, however, rediscovered and during a long period of peace, brought about by Emperor Charlemagne and his armies, the church was rebuilt. A service of rededication to St Anne was held in 792AD. Charlemagne attended the service. The congregation was large and at the front stood a boy of fourteen who had been blind, deaf, and dumb since birth. During the service he became agitated and tap-tapping his stick made his way to the altar. He indicated that a flagstone at the foot of the altar should be lifted.

Below the flagstone was a passageway with a door at the end – before the astonished eyes of the congregation the door opened spontaneously to reveal a crypt lit by a single lamp burning brightly in a niche. The lamp's rays illuminated a casket resting on the earthen floor in the middle of the crypt. The lid of the casket was removed and beneath was a shroud which was clearly labelled as containing the remains of St Anne – at the very moment of revelation the lamp flame guttered, and died – and the boy could speak, hear, and see.

BACK TO THE PROVENCE-BOUND SHIPLOAD OF NAZARENES: the Divine Hand had not guided the boat directly to the coast of France, on the way it called at Alexandria where a dark-skinned, Egyptian Christian serving girl, Sarah, was waiting. Sarah had begged to be allowed to join the boat but somehow managed to miss the sailing time. No matter, in that age of miracles, she was able to board the boat as it stood offshore. First she walked on the water and then when she got close to the boat one of the passengers, Mary Salomé, cast her cloak into the sea where it turned into a raft. Sarah stood on the raft and when it floated alongside she was able to clamber up the side and board the boat.

The boat's manifest included the three sainted Marys who were the first to witness Jesus' empty tomb after the Resurrection – St Mary Salomé (mother of James and John), St Mary Jacobi (sister or cousin of the Virgin Mary) and St Mary Magdalene, who was accompanied by her sister, Martha, and her brother, Lazarus – again confusion

– some say the sister of Martha and Lazarus was Mary of Bethany and not Mary Magdalene.

Lazarus was very much alive but depressed. After his resurrection Lazarus never smiled. He had been dead for four days when Jesus performed the miracle of his resurrection and during that time he had viewed existence in the after-life. He never spoke of it but evidently had been filled with dread by what he had seen.

Some accounts indicate that there were fourteen bishops on the boat while others state that only three disciples, St Simon, St Maximin, and St Philip were among the passengers. Saint Simon, the Cyrene, was the passer-by who was forced by Roman soldiers to help Jesus carry the cross (years later St Simon had a son, St Ruf, who became the first bishop of Avignon). The second disciple, St Maximin, became the first Bishop of Aix-en-Provence. His most distinguished act came about some thirty years later when he administered extreme unction to St Mary Magadalene. The third disciple was St Philip the Evangelist.

In another account, Philip the Evangelist had arrived ahead of the boat and was waiting on the shore. He greeted the saintly passengers as the boat beached and as they disembarked St Philip instructed Joseph of Arimethea not to linger but to continue on his journey. He told Joseph to travel on to the north of France and cross the Channel to St Michael's Mount in Cornwall; where he was to begin his mission of converting the Britons, starting with the Cornish Celts.

The boat had reached France at the delta of the river Rhône on the coast of the Camargue and where its passengers disembarked a town sprang up. In time it was, appropriately, called Les Saintes Mairies de la Mer (The Sainted Marys from the Sea) and became the capital of the Camargue.

As soon as the passengers were disembarked they started preaching and converting the locals, including the occupying Romans, to Christianity. Sarah, the dark-skinned Egyptian, went preaching and begging through the Camargue. Centuries later gypsies adopted her as their patron saint. On her feast day, 24 May, the effigy of Sarah, the Black Madonna, is taken from the church and paraded through the streets of Saintes Mairies de la Mer. The day-long ceremony concludes with horsemen on white Camargue horses carrying St Sarah to the beach for a splash through the waves before returning her to repose in the town church for another year.

Two of the Marys, Salomé and Jacobi, were elderly and saw out their days at Saintes Mairies de la Mer. St Martha settled near Avignon and converted the local population to Christianity. By all accounts she was a nice, gentle lady, always anxious to please. Her story in the Bible began when Jesus called at her home in the fishing town of Magdala on the shore of Lake Galilee. It was a wealthy home, Simon the Pharisee was the owner and father of Martha, her sister Mary and her brother Lazarus. Martha prepared a meal while Jesus and sister, Mary, talked matters spiritual.

It has to be remarked that there is confusion as to the true identity of the Mary who sat at Jesus' feet. Was she Mary Magdalene or was she Mary Bethany or was she a third Mary, of low repute, who happened to walk into the house of Simon the Pharisee? Roman Catholic tradition conflated all the Marys into one person, Pope Saint Gregory the Great (540-604AD) officially identified Mary Bethany and Mary Magdalene as one person in the 6th century and this declaration lasted to the early 1900s. This resolved the confusion caused by the Saints Jerome, Augustine, Albertus Magnus, and Thomas Aquinas, all of whom had been unable to make a decision as to which Mary was the true Magdalene.

No matter whichever, the story goes that before dinner Mary washed the feet of Jesus with her tears, dried them with her long flowing hair and then poured a jar of expensive, perfumed ointment over them. Meanwhile Martha was doing the cooking; she was later adopted as the patron saint of servants and cooks.

Martha's most celebrated act in Provence was to see to the destruction of a monster which lived in the river Rhône at Tarascon, a town near Avignon. The ancient town is still there with its magnificent castle beautifully restored and mirrored in the slow waters of the broad river. The monster, known as the Tarasque, was fearsome; it had the head of a lion, its body was half beast and half fish and it had wings like a dragon with a tail like a serpent. The Tarasque was immensely strong and impossible to kill because of an extraordinary defence mechanism – if chased it would spread its ordure over an area the size of an acre and it was powerful stuff – reflecting light like glass and anything it touched would burst into flames. The Tarasque had a nasty habit of leaping out of hiding places on the river bank and seizing and eating passers-by, with a penchant for children. The Tarasque also enjoyed sinking any boats which came within its reach.

One day the locals went to Martha while she was at prayer and told her of the monster's latest activities. She instantly declared that she would help and at the head of a great throng came upon the Tarasque in the woods finishing off a half-eaten child. Martha sprinkled the monster with holy water from her cook's ladle. The Tarasque was immobilised but to make sure she bound it with the girdle of her dress. Despite the Tarasque's legendary strength, of twelve lions, the monster found itself unable to move and the throng cheerfully killed it with spears and swords, before tearing it to pieces.

At eighty years of age Martha died in Tarascon and was buried there. But intervention by her on behalf of Christians was called upon again fifteen centuries later. Berber pirates were on the point of attacking Villajoyosa in Spain when their fleet was destroyed by a flash flood; which was attributed, for reasons arcane, to Martha.

If there is a ranking order the most important St Mary next to the Virgin Mary, and the one with the most legends and cult theories attached to her name, is Mary Magdalene. What is alleged to be her true story is that at first she went from Saintes Mairies de la Mer to Marseille, where she preached the Gospel. Whilst preaching she encountered the Prince and Princess of Marseille making sacrifices to a pagan god in the hope that their barren marriage would be blessed with a child. Mary instructed them to cease worshipping pagan gods and told them that she would intercede with God on their behalf. She did and they had a child. The grateful Prince converted to Christianity. He had every pagan temple in Marseille destroyed and replaced by a Christian church. Much later, in the twelfth century, it was recounted that the Prince and his Princess made Mary Magdalene's brother, Lazarus, the first bishop of Marseille.

After converting the whole of Provence Mary Magdalene retired to a cave on a hillside overlooking Marseille and there she spent her final thirty years in prayer and fasting. She took no food at all but she survived because every day at noon a group of angels descended and took her to heaven where she was nourished by the Holy Eucharist. The ascent was witnessed and verified by a shepherd. St Mary Magdalene died at the age of seventy-two. In her final hours she was taken by angels to a chapel in Aix-en-Provence where Bishop St Maximin administered the last rites.

BUT ALTERNATIVE VERSIONS GIVE DIFFERENT ACCOUNTS OF the life of Mary Magdalene. Enter Dan Brown, the Da Vinci code, the Abbé of Rennes le Château, and the Gnostics… the possessors of hidden knowledge. All have a common thread – Jesus did not die on the cross and he was married… married to Mary Magdalene

Most of the stories hinge on the theory that although

Jesus appeared to die fact he became deeply sedated after
he being given, on a stick, a sponge soaked in a liquid to
suck. The liquid was said to have been vinegar, but it was
not, it was a strong solution of an opiate and he was thus
able to leave the tomb when the effects of the narcotic
wore off.

The alternative theorists also maintain that Jesus and
Mary Magdalene were married, the marriage had taken
place at Cana – the groom provided the wine, six hundred
litres of it. They, and daughter Sara, were among the
passengers on the boat which landed at Sainte Mairies de la
Mer. The accounts are vague concerning what happened
after they landed but it was said that from the Camargue,
when Mary went to Marseille, Jesus followed her and then
they journeyed to Rennes-les-Bains in the Aude, three
kilometres from where a village called Rennes-le-Chateau
would appear later. They settled in Rennes-les-Bains and
had more children; their descendants married into the
Merovingian dynasty and walk among us to this day.

The Merovingians are a fertile source of awe for those
desperate to believe in the weird and wonderful. Believers
regard the line as beginning in Egypt thirteen centuries
before Christ, that the bloodline has been passed down
through the centuries and exists to this day. During the
aeons of the passage of time the bloodline has included
celebrities as diverse as the Pharaohs, Queen Cleopatra,
Alexander the Great, and the Emperor Constantine. With
the collapse of Rome the Merovingians formed the first
royal dynasty of France. Merovingians trace the bloodline
of James the First, King of England, back to the pharaohs
and forward to modern times, to the British royal family,
the House of Windsor. Presidents of the United States,
from George Washington to George Bush all carried the
line and no doubt some connection to the Merovingians
can be attributed to Mr Barack Obama.

Abbé Bérenger Saunière (1852-1917), the parish priest
of Rennes-le-Chateau was said to prefer wine and women

to his priestly duties. Out of the blue and with no explanation the Abbé became rich. He restored his parish church, already dedicated to St Mary Magdalene, built a tower and a library. He adopted a wealthy lifestyle and enjoyed even more frequent bawdy parties.

It was rumoured that his sudden wealth came from blackmailing the Roman Catholic Church to the tune of twenty-eight million pieces of gold, and that he was able to do so because he had discovered the tombs of Jesus and Mary Magdalene. Alternatively, that he had found the marriage certificate of Jesus and Mary, written on ancient papyrus. Publication of either story would destroy dogma essential to the Church of Rome.

Over the years many fruitless searches for the tomb have been made in Rennes-le-Chateau. The occupying Nazi Germans in World War II dug over much of the village; the only hitherto-unknown grave they found contained three skeletons with bullet holes in their skulls.

PERHAPS, HOWEVER, THE ABBÉ SAUNIERE'S ABILITY to blackmail the Church had nothing to do with the discovery of tombs at Rennes-le-Chateau and maybe Jesus was buried elsewhere. Twenty years ago my wife and I, while visiting Kashmir, were taken to the back streets of downtown Srinagar to see the 'real tomb' of Jesus. It was in a tumbledown wooden hut with green and white peeling paint and festooned, as was the whole of Srinagar, with electric power lines which sagged dangerously, in this case within a couple of inches of the tin roof of the hut. I asked the attendant, 'How do you know that this is the tomb of Jesus?'

He replied, 'Jesus big man, this big tomb.'

He then pointed to an nearby large marble slab with a depression on the surface, which could with a little imagination be interpreted as a large footprint.

'That Jesus footprint, it big foot print,' then adding triumphantly and conclusively, 'Jesus big man, big feet.'

Then, confidentially, 'Jesus come again… and when he come again… he come Srinagar.'

Another saintly passenger, St Joseph of Arimathea, the great uncle of Jesus, was aboard the boat and was sent to Britain; he had been before. He was a rich man, a successful tin merchant; maybe he obtained his supplies of tin, like the Phoenicians had for centuries, from Cornwall, in the southwest of Britain. At the time of the crucifixion he donated what was destined to be his own tomb for the body of Christ. He supplied the winding sheets and oils for the preparation of the corpse. He acquired the cup used by Jesus at The Last Supper. At the crucifixion when, towards the end, a Roman soldier speared Jesus in the side, Joseph held out the cup to receive the blood and fluid which exuded from the wound. That simple cup was then transmuted into the sacred chalice which became known as the Holy Grail… the symbol of ultimate spiritual perfection.

Joseph's story, like so many saintly tales, is chronologically confusing. According to some in his first visit to what was to become the south of England he was accompanied by the boy Jesus. Centuries later this was hinted at in 'Jerusalem,' a hymn nearly as dear to the English as their National Anthem. William Blake's eighteenth century words tell of building a New Jerusalem among England's 'dark, satanic mills' – referring to the Industrial Revolution, or perhaps to the universities of Oxford and Cambridge. We still wait for the New Jerusalem, nearly all the dark satanic mills have long disappeared and the Oxbridge Universities, while having a reputation of elitism, have no suggestion of Satanism about them.

Uncle Joseph and the boy Jesus built a daub-and-wattle church at Glastonbury and according to legend (during Joseph's subsequent visit following the crucifixion) Joseph buried the Holy Grail in England. Sir Thomas Malory (died 1471, aged about 55), thief, rapist, extortionist, bandit, kidnapper, and Member of Parliament spent many years in jail where he wrote his chef d'oeuvre, 'Le Morte d'Arthur.' In it he tells of the chivalry of the Knights of the Round Table and recounts how King Arthur and his entourage never found the Holy Grail despite spending scores of knight-years in the search.

WHILE MONTPELLIER, FIFTY KILOMETRES TO THE WEST of Saintes Maries de la Mer, was attracting Arab scholars from the Eastern Mediterranean and establishing the first university in Europe, Marseille eighty kilometres to the east of Montpellier, was busy importing plague-infected fleas on the backs of rats from the Levant.

The first recorded outbreak of La Peste, the Black Death, in Marseilles occurred in the 6th century AD. Eight hundred years later, in just one outbreak, it killed twenty-five million across Europe. There were repeated outbreaks over succeeding years and in 1720 the Great Plague of Marseille killed a hundred thousand in the city and the same number in the surrounding region. The origin of this episode is clear; several members of the crew of a merchant ship, including the ship's surgeon, died of the plague during a voyage from the Levant. On arrival in Marseilles the port authorities promptly put the ship in quarantine. But powerful city merchants, who owned the boat's cargo of silks and cottons, successfully pressed the authorities to lift the quarantine. A few days later plague broke out in the city. The huge number of deaths rapidly overwhelmed the city's public health services and thousands of bloated, blackened corpses lay scattered individually and in piles around the city.

The Black Death arrives in two main forms, bubonic and pneumonic with less commonly, a septicaemic form. Pneumonic plague kills quickly, sometimes so quickly that the victim literally drops dead. Pneumonic plague is airborne and enters via the lungs where it causes a fulminant, haemorrhagic pneumonia. Sufferers turn black because they are deeply cyanosed. Their blood is almost black in colour and as venous blood flows through the lungs the extensive pneumonia prevents oxygen reaching the blood to turn it to the normal bright red colour of arterial blood.

The bubonic form kills less quickly but it is a horrible, painful death. Large abscesses, called buboes, form in the lymph nodes and elsewhere. Bleeding into the kidneys produces black urine, bleeding into the gut produces black stools and bleeding beneath the skin produces black areas which coalesce and can make the victim appear entirely black.

To prevent the spread of the plague from Marseilles the parliament at Aix passed a law which inflicted the death penalty on persons who left the city during an epidemic. The desperately frightened authorities built a wall, two metres high and guarded by troops, surrounding Marseilles to prevent human plague carriers leaving.

The plague spread rapidly and logical measures like the mass killing of Jews and self-flagellation, did not work. What was needed was an antibiotic which would kill Yersinia pestis (formerly Pasteurella pestis), the plague bacteria; but the world would have to wait another quarter of a millennium for that. Meanwhile the population took the only action they could, they appealed for divine help.

To the north west of Mont Ventoux lies the valley of St Sebastian, the original plague saint. In it stands a small statue of the young St Sebastian. Originally his trunk was pierced with arrows but in recent years children pulled them out to play with, and naturally they were lost. Not far away is a simple chapel dedicated to St Roch, the other specialist plague saint. Small chapels, dedicated to Saints Roch and Sebastian, punctuate the roads of Provence. In plague epidemics (real or rumoured) processions of the fearful faithful prayed in those chapels for an end to the Black Death. Both saints were home-grown French;

Sebastian was born in Narbonne and Roch in Montpellier.

St Sebastian (martyred about 288AD) was originally a locally enlisted Roman soldier. He rose to the rank of captain in the Praetorian Guard but he embraced Christianity. Sebastian fell foul of the authorities when in Rome, during the great persecution of Christians by Emperor Diocletian, he persuaded Christian prisoners to hold firmly onto their faith. On the Emperor's instructions fellow Roman soldiers took him to a field, tied him to a post, shot his body full of arrows, and left him for dead.

His body was taken by a widow, Irene of Rome, and prepared for burial, but discovering that he was still alive she nursed him back to health. After he had convalesced, Sebastian, while sitting on a veranda, spotted Diocletian passing by being carried on a litter. Sebastian harangued the Emperor for his paganism. Diocletian recognised him and promptly ordered a platoon of Roman soldiers to take him back to that same field where he had been shot full of arrows and club him to death, making sure this time that he really was dead. Sebastian became known as The Double Martyr and was admitted to the Roll of the Saints of Rome. In 1348 Europe was ravaged by the Black Death. In their terror supplicants en masse offered prayers to St Sebastian – miraculously the epidemic was halted.

At the time of his martyrdom Sebastian was a grizzled, middle-aged man, but from 1000AD many artists depicted him as Oscar Wilde much later described him as, 'A lovely brown boy with crisp, clustering hair and red lips.'

TODAY'S GAYS HAVE ADOPTED HIM AS AN ICON. A Japanese writer, Yukio Mishima, a sado-masochism enthusiast, wrote, 'His martyrdom symbolised the erotic pleasure of pain.' Finally, in a grand gesture of his solidarity with Sebastian, Mishima dressed up as a Saint Sebastian look-alike, had his photograph taken, and then ritually disembowelled himself.

Despite Oscar Wilde's drooling description there is no

evidence that Sebastian was gay. Contemporary gay activists lobbied the Papacy to add 'gay' to his entry in the Calendar of Saints, but Pope John Paul II side-stepped that plea. Sebastian is named on the Roll of Saints as the patron saint of plague victims; the dying, municipal workers, and the police.

Saint Roch's father was a nobleman and governor of Montpellier. His wife was barren; she prayed to the Virgin Mary, her prayers were rewarded. She fell pregnant and delivered a healthy boy whom they christened Roch. The baby had a red birthmark in the shape of a crucifix on the front of his chest; it remained there throughout his life and was to be the means of identifying him after death. It was probably a cavernous haemangioma, commonly called a port-wine stain.

St Roch's parents died when he was twenty. He inherited the Governorship of Montpellier but handed it over to an uncle. He gave all his worldly possessions to the poor and early in the fourteenth century, on foot, took the road to Rome as a mendicant pilgrim.

St Roch encountered cases of the plague and cured them by prayer and making a sign of the cross on the sufferer. Eventually he himself became ill, presumably with the plague. He took himself to a forest where miraculously a spring of sweet water sprang up where he lay down. A Count's hunting dog came upon him and every day for many weeks brought him bread and licked his wounds until they healed.

Eventually St Roch returned to Montpellier, incognito. He was arrested as a spy and thrown in jail by his Uncle's men. He languished there for five years without disclosing his identity, but it was revealed when he died and the cruciform birthmark on his chest was seen. Soon after he died an angel came to his cell and placed under his head a tablet on which was written in letters of gold, 'who calleth meekly to Saint Roch he shall not be hurt with any hurt of the pestilence.'

THE FRENCH HAVE A SPECIAL WORD FOR BEHEADED SAINTS who carried their heads – céphalophores. It is said that one hundred and thirty have existed in France. One was St Mitre (433-466AD) who was a Greek immigrant field worker in Aix-en-Provence. He upset his Roman master by openly criticising his morals, the master was living with a wife, but she was not his own. One day the boss was told that Mitre had stolen his entire grape harvest. He confronted Mitre and accused him of the theft, but when he inspected his vineyards he found that all his vines were intact and bearing sweet, plump, grapes. Naturally he charged Mitre with sorcery, declared him guilty and had him beheaded in the city square. Mitre immediately picked up his head and walked to the church in Aix where he placed it on the altar and then expired. For many years St Mitre's tombstone discharged a liquid, through a shining hole, which cured eye sores.

Another céphalophore, St Aphrodise, while preaching on a camel in Béziers was seized and beheaded by pagans. His head was thrown into a well which instantly gushed water so forcefully that the head was ejected. Whereupon Aphrodise picked it up and, continuing preaching, carried his head to the local church and laid it on the altar. In the third century St Just, a boy of nine, was also seized and beheaded while preaching. Following céphalophore custom he held his head in his hands and continued to preach, expiring at the end of his sermon.

How many French saints are there? Impossible to say without a great deal of research but inspection of French place names beginning with Saint, or the feminine Sainte, in the Michelin guide shows about five thousand. For what it's worth, the ratio is ten male saints to one female sainte. And how many saints are there? According to the Book of Revelations they are too numerous to count – I hope that there is still enough room in heaven for the likes of you and me.

16. THE GREAT RETURN

THE FRENCH ARE CREATURES OF HABIT, particularly when it comes to mealtimes. Lunch is from noon onwards, the length of the lunch hour depends on who or what you are. If you are a tourist and you turn up at half past one, at best you will get a frosty reception and a cold, 'installez vous' as you are directed to a table next to the swinging kitchen door; the worst, 'nous n'avons pas une table,' when you can clearly see two or three empty tables before your eyes. If you book an evening meal and you turn up between seven and eight the table is yours for the evening but if you haven't booked and appear after nine you may be brusquely turned away, as my wife and I were from an almost empty restaurant.

The French love to chat. At the check-out in the supermarché if the cashier is an acquaintance of the customer ahead, you can expect to wait while pleasantries and news are exchanged, no matter how long the queue. When driving the French habitually tail-gate believing it is friendly but dawdling on your part has to be deliberate provocation and demands an angry hoot. If on a country road two drivers ahead, travelling in opposite directions, have stopped, blocked the road and are hanging out of their windows engaged in conversation it is very rude to honk them. They will still take their time, they won't budge, and if you continuously thump your horn you'll get angry stares and often a gesture involving the middle finger.

We had been residing in France for six months before the September Rentrée, the Great French Return, happened. I had heard about it from my French teacher, Hervé, at Alliance Française, the French Cultural Institute, where we took French lessons when we lived in Dubai.

Hervé was a delightful young man and a good teacher of French. He would enliven such mind-numbing subjects as the various forms of the subjunctive with intriguing tales of the peculiarities of French life, la vie française, for the benefit of those in his class (like me) who intended to make their homes in France. One piece of whimsy I remember was *le croque-mort*. I already knew that a croque-monsieur was a toasted ham and cheese sandwich and if you stuck a fried egg on top it became a croque-madame, but croque-mort? Croquer means to bite into, to crunch – like Adam biting or croqueing into Eve's crunchy offering – but mort, dead? What's a dead toasted sandwich? With a smile Hervé explained.

In bygone days, after the priest had administered the last rites and the undertaker appeared the first thing he did was to grasp one of the corpse's legs, raise the foot to his mouth and bite hard into the big toe joint; a highly sensitive and tender spot. No reaction confirmed that that the deceased really had departed. Croque-mort has an informality which is less daunting than the standard French for undertaker – un entrepreneur des pompes funèbres.

My wife and I had enrolled at the Alliance Française because we had bought a tumble-down property in sunny Provence and planned to retire there in a couple of years. After twenty-five years in the sunshine of the Middle East, the cool, wet climate of England did not appeal; leave alone a society which had developed terminal political correctness and an inability of TV writers to sling together half a dozen words without using the 'F' word.

With regret I quit Hervé's enjoyable sessions because I had a brainwave – I would teach English to the French in my small town. I knew the French were desperate to learn English to join the proper world. I needed a qualification so I enrolled in a six month TESOL (Teaching English to Speakers of Other Languages) course in Dubai.

THE SECOND SURPRISE, AFTER I HAD WRITTEN A SURPRISINGLY LARGE CHEQUE, was that I was the only bloke in a class of thirteen and I was old enough to be a grandfather to half the girls. I was startled yet again, half way through the first lesson.

We had enjoyed a coffee break and I had taken advantage of what both the French and the English call the WC. I was settling in my chair when a particularly aggressive (and somewhat spotty) young lady stood, reddened and addressed the teacher, 'Would you please tell members of the class to lower the toilet seat after use!'

Naturally all eyes swivelled towards me, I was the only one with an inherent standing advantage – I said nothing, what could I do but gaze around appearing both mystified and innocent. But whenever the need again arose, as I left, I would make darned sure that the seat was defiantly vertical.

Looking back on it, my English teaching career in France could not have been described as… distinguished. For starters, I soon found that those ungrateful French were not falling over themselves for my services – adverts in the local supermarkets attracted no attention – I ended up mostly teaching sixteen-year-old daughters of French acquaintances, pas mal. My earnings in the course of two years amounted to two bottles of red wine, a stuffed guinea fowl, and one hundred and fifty euros.

I was invited to teach in the Lien Social as one of a

group of volunteers who in the evenings would teach children who were having difficulties with a particular subject at school. The parents were enthusiastic, it was free, but the children were not interested... after all, being not interested was what made them no good. It was uphill for me – I worked harder than any three students combined. The final straw came in the form of a very pleasant, smiling, ten year old imp, who had an amazing talent. He could fart, loud and long, seemingly at will. Each time he exploded the class collapsed – and so did I – how could I exercise authority with tears streaming down my face?

Maybe I would have done better in Dubai to forget TESOL and stick with Hervé; after all it was from him that I learned so much useful local knowledge, like for instance when he once told us, 'If you want to post a parcel, don't do it in June – the French are thinking of going on strike; don't do it in July – they are on strike and don't do it in August – they are on holiday, wait until September, everything starts with a bang, everything works because then it's La Rentrée.'

UNTIL WE CAME TO FRANCE I HAD NO IDEA OF THE MASSIVE significance of La Rentrée. France is a secular country, but you could be forgiven for thinking La Rentrée heralded the second coming of the Messiah. Shops, supermarkets, newspapers, and ladies' magazines are full of advertisements for La Rentrée, and the town buzzes with parents discussing plans for their children's Rentrée Scolaire.

Ideally you should finish your year's work by the end of May, leaving enough time to wind down to take your deserved holiday in August. The French work an exhausting thirty-five hour week, have a couple of bank holidays each month, and if it happens that they fall on a Thursday or Tuesday it is only right for them to attach the intervening Friday or Monday to the weekend and so have several four-day breaks each year. In the run-up to the universal August vacations fonctionnaires (civil servants) fill their pending trays, roofers stop roofing… there might be hidden wasps nests, and vignerons can relax while the sun obligingly tops up the sugar in their grapes and they top up their energy in preparation for the mad dash of the vendange, the wine harvest, in September.

For a couple of weeks before La Rentrée, the French version of Amazon, Amazon.fr, ever mindful of my needs, bombards me with suggestions that I should profit by their offer of une rentrée scolaire sans stress, toutes les fournitures scolaire – no stress and everything needed for the school return – everything but everything, from satchel to crayons, from pencil sharpener to glue, all in a job-lot to make sure that little Jean-Paul has everything he needs for his rentrée scolaire.

FORTUNATELY FOR ME AT THIS TIME I AM calmness personified. I have no job; I am retired and long past the stresses of raising children. While the whole of France, adults and schoolchildren, are frantic about La Rentrée, for my personal Rentrée I think a dive in the swimming pool and a glass of Côtes du Rhône Villages rouge will do the trick.

17. VINCENT AND THE GREEN FAIRY

DOES ABSINTHE MAKE THE HEART GROW FONDER? Seems it did for Vincent van Gogh.

Vincent van Gogh was one of the great impressionist artists who moved to Provence to capture its extraordinary light and ambience. He rented a house in the Provençal town of Arles. The house was yellow and his paintings of it survive, but the house itself was destroyed by Allied bombing in World War II.

One Christmas he invited a fellow artist, Paul Gauguin, to stay with him and together they would paint. Vincent was an unstable character with a history of unpredictable behaviour, especially when tanked-up with alcohol. In one violent episode Vincent inexplicably cut off his right ear. Although details vary, it is likely that the most reliable account of van Gogh's ear auto-amputation can be found in the contemporary local newspapers. From several it appears that one evening, just before Christmas in 1888, after a few days on the absinthe, he quarrelled with Paul Gauguin. During the quarrel the befuddled Vincent opened a cut-throat razor and sliced off all but the lobe of his left ear, nicking the nearby posterior auricular artery.

Gauguin fled. Van Gogh wrapped the bloody object in

newspaper and clutching it, fell out through the door of his yellow house. He tottered down the street to his local brothel (Maison de Tolérance no: 1), and knocked on the door, it was opened by Rachel, a servant girl. He knew and admired her, they were good friends. Vincent handed her the bloody parcel saying, 'Keep this object carefully.'

Then turning on his heel he staggered back to his yellow house, lay down on his rickety yellow bed and descended into a deep absinthe-sedated sleep.

Rachel screamed and fainted when she opened Vincent's grisly parcel. Later, that evening, she went to the Gendarmerie and handed the blood-soaked object to the duty policeman, probably saying something like, 'That ginger-headed lunatic of a painter gave me this.'

The policeman instantly knew who she was talking about. Vincent had been reported many times after townswomen had complained of his behaviour; in fact all the citizens of Arles knew him and called him 'le fou roux' - the crazy redhead. The duty gendarme put the horrible package to one side.

The following morning, while he was presenting his night report, he showed the bloody package to his boss, the inspector. Sensing something serious was up the inspector ordered the gendarme to accompany him and together they rushed to van Gogh's house. The inspector ordered the gendarme to knock down the locked front door and they dashed upstairs to find a barely conscious Vincent lying on his blood-soaked bed.

He was admitted as an emergency to l'Hôtel Dieu, the local hospital in Arles. He survived the wound; survived the doctors, and survived the hospital. A blessing for the world, for after he recovered his output of paintings was enormous.

Vincent subsequently had two episodes of being so disturbed that he had to be admitted to the Saint Paul Asylum in Saint-Rémy-de-Provence, but even when committed to that mental hospital he continued to paint prodigiously.

Eighteen months later, on 29 July 1890, Vincent van Gogh died and his tormented life ended. The circumstances of his death remain confused. Contemporary reports varied –. some said that he had shot himself in the chest, others that he had shot himself in the abdomen. Some say deliberately by his own hand, others that he was shot accidentally by the hand of a young boy who was playing nearby with a loaded pistol. The true story will never be known.

The tragic fate of van Gogh is known, but what happened to the ear he chopped off in December 1888? The police gave it to Dr Félix Rey, his physician in the Hôtel Dieu. Dr Rey put it in a jar of formalin and forgot it. He lost the jar when he moved to Paris a few years later.

WHAT A PRIZE IF THAT PICKLED PINNA HAD SURVIVED? Maybe it is still lurking, a ghostly white ear floating in a dust covered jar of formalin at the back of some shelf – it could now be worth as much as the eighty million US dollars paid at Christie's New York auction house in 1990 by a Japanese industrial-paper tycoon for van Gogh's portrait of his physician, Dr Gachet. That was one of his last paintings and was never seen again after the Japanese tycoon had paid for it. Within days the painting was crated and sent to Tokyo – rumour has it that the painting was cremated, along with his corpse when the tycoon died six years later in 1996.

Scientists in Boston have, however, made a living replica of van Gogh's ear using genetic material taken from the great-great grandson of Vincent's brother Theo. It is alive! Kept in a nutrient solution it houses a microphone into which one can speak, with what in mind, and with no possibility of a response, the exercise seems pointless. Perhaps a sympathetic scientist has pickled it in absinthe.

So can we say that it was absinthe which made Vincent

yearn to give Rachel a token of his affection? And why did he choose his left ear? The answer to the second question is simple, he was right handed. There is no simple answer to the first question. Perhaps, of the many theories put forward over the years, the most plausible is that the absinthe-befuddled Vincent was simply imitating the events and the actions of the local heroes, the matadors, in the Arles bullfights.

In the Arles bullring, built originally as a Roman amphitheatre, after a difficult, but elegantly executed kill of a particularly aggressive and cunning bull, the President of La Féria, prompted by an excited crowd, would wave a white handkerchief signalling that he would award one of the bull's ears to the matador. The young, brave, handsome, and skilled matador dressed in his colourful, skin-tight livery would step up, proudly accept the honour and then, with a gallant flourish, present the ear to the lady of his choice. One, perhaps dubious, hypothesis is that Vincent presented his ear to Rachel symbolizing – *I am the bull, and Rachel, you are my conquering matador.*

ABSINTHE IS A STRONG GREEN SPIRIT made with a base of fifty-five per cent distilled ethyl alcohol. Aniseed gives the dominant flavour and subtle flavours are added by the herbs; wormwood, hyssop and melissa; all of which provide chlorophyll to make the colour green. An early form of absinthe was popular with sailors in the Middle Ages. It was a wormwood-based drink taken for its medicinal properties – it soothed sore throats, relieved toothache and cured seasickness… it also got rid of fleas.

Early in its history absinthe developed a reputation for stimulating both thought and sexual prowess, hence its appeal to the Bohemian ways of artists and intellectuals like Toulouse Lautrec, Oscar Wilde, Picasso, Hemingway, and celebrities like Franklin D. Roosevelt and Frank Sinatra. Alas, those effects are illusory, as is the effect that absinthe in large quantities can induce a sense of extreme mental clarity and an ability to think with amazing insight. As for its alleged aphrodisiac qualities, these are simply related to the alcohol content and alcohol, as Shakespeare said, 'provoketh the desire,' and – one might surmise, from personal experience – added the corollary, 'but taketh away the performance.'

Towards the end of the eighteenth century a French doctor in Switzerland, Dr Pierre Ordinaire, produced an Elixir of Absinthe. On his death his housekeeper sold the doctor's recipe which then passed through several hands until in 1797, it was bought by a certain Major Dubied who with his son-in-law, Henri-Luis Pernod, founded the first commercial absinthe making establishment at Couvet in Switzerland.

The French quickly became avid consumers of absinthe but imported from Switzerland it attracted custom duties. Messieurs Dubied and Pernod side-stepped those by transferring their factory to France... no import duty, cheap absinthe, and an enthusiastic public made it even more popular.

THE RAPID ASCENT OF ABSINTHE WAS ASSURED, so rapid that in 1850 the President of The French League against Alcohol, lamented, 'France drinks more absinthe than the rest of the world put together.'

French consumption reached 7,000 hectolitres (150,000 gallons) by 1874 and 360,000 hectolitres (nearly eight million gallons) twenty five years later. A journalist at that time wrote, 'The whole world drinks absinthe; from the hotel porter, whose doctor recommended it for his weak stomach, to the brilliant, street-smart bourgeoisie.'

Absinthe became so fashionable that bottle labels reflected contemporary life. The brand La Pedalette marked the first commercial appearance of the bicycle. Popular postcards depicting generously-busted maidens were sold in their thousands; they proclaimed absinthe's benefits: TONIQUE, HYGIENIQUE, GAIE – POUR

183

CONSERVER LE VIGUEUR!

In 1895 the Dreyfus Affair provoked a powerful wave of anti-Semitism in France. Alfred Dreyfus was a Jewish artillery captain in the French army who had been accused of treason; court-martialled, found guilty and condemned to be sent to Devil's Island which is a notorious, disease-ridden penitentiary on a tropical island, fourteen kilometres off the coast of the French colony of Guyana in South America. It is surrounded by brutally dangerous waters and escape from it has always been well-nigh impossible.

The larger absinthe manufacturers, themselves Jewish and widely known to be so, were alarmed; their commercial anxiety outweighed any other sentiments and they promptly labelled their bottles – 'Absinthe Anti-Juive. France aux Français!' – Anti-Jewish Absinthe - France for the French!

After six year's solitary confinement and untiring efforts by his wife, Lucie, to have his name cleared, his lawyers presented evidence of conspiracy and fraud. It took two retrials before Dreyfus was declared innocent. He resumed his army career and the Jewish absinthe makers relabelled their bottles.

In the 1840s, to prevent malaria, French army doctors gave absinthe to the troops fighting in Algeria. It appeared to be effective, but how did it work? Perhaps when the female anopheles mosquito imbibed a proboscis-full of absinthe-laden blood she would topple off her perch before being able to inject her victim with a load of malarial parasites. Or, maybe those doctors knew a thing or two or, had unwittingly hit on a rational treatment.

Since 350BC the Chinese have used an extract of the leaves of the plant, Artemesia annua (sweet wormwood), closely related to Artemesia absinthium (the variety named for its use in making absinthe) to treat malaria.

Nowadays, Western Medicine is using the same extract

of the annua variety, called artemesinin, to successfully treat cases of the most deadly form of the disease, falciparum malaria. Whether those military doctors knew about the Chinese traditional treatment is not known, but, sure as night follows day, the French soldiers acquired a taste for absinthe.

Absinthe became an icon of La Vie Bohème and so popular in bistros, bars and cafés that in the 1860s the hour of five o'clock in the afternoon was called l'Heure Verte, the Green Hour.

EVERYWHERE PEOPLE 'SOAKED THEIR ABSINTHE' in a ceremony which had become an art. Habitués would pour 30mls of the green absinthe into a special glass, then resting a perforated or slotted spoon, holding a cube or two of sugar, across the mouth of the glass would gently trickle 150mls of iced water through the sugar. Soon swirling shapes and faint fairy-like figures would appear in a milky fog. Devotees knew how to make la fée (the fairy) appear and by turning and twisting the glass promote the release of subtle perfumes. Of course, one had to be patient and appreciate that the fairy might not appear until at least the third glass had been drunk. The bourgeoisie had nothing but contempt for those peasants who ignored the art and simply topped the green liquor with water, swished it around and swigged it down.

Anyone who has drunk pastis or ouzo knows that when you add water to the undiluted, clear liquor it becomes cloudy. This is because these liquors, which resemble absinthe, contain plant substances called terpenoids, distant cousins of turpentine. Terpenoids are held in solution by a high concentration of alcohol. When the concentration is reduced, by the addition of water, the terpenoids come out of solution to form a whitish-yellow opalescence.

The clarity of the original liquor can be restored very simply by returning the alcohol content to its original concentration of 55%, by the addition of a few shots of neat spirit. Drinking such a powerful potion is not recommended; for obvious reasons. One habitué, the artist Toulouse-Lautrec, routinely added brandy to his absinthe; but in his case, because of his short, crippled legs, he did not have far to fall.

Absinthe contains, in addition to terpenoids, another chemical called thujone, it is related to menthol and derived from the essential oils of wormwood. It was the thujone which gave absinthe its evil reputation. The acute toxic effects of thujone include; convulsions, visual and auditory hallucinations, and in the long-term, brain damage, psychiatric illness and suicidal tendencies. The French doctors of the era of van Gogh distinguished l'absinthisme as an illness distinct from l'alcoolisme.

Absinthe became popular internationally but no country's consumption exceeded that of France. Priests complained that many of the population not working on a Sunday would not attend Holy Mass but spend the Sabbath Day in taverns, which called themselves cafeterias.. In 1850 the ratio was 330,000 cafeterias to 30,000 churches.

Priests were up in arms and sober citizens were alarmed by large numbers of drunks tottering along the roads, so much so that owners of carriages would not drive on Sundays and feast days for fear of running down staggering pedestrians. A turning point came in 1905 when a certain Swiss man, Jean Lanfray, murdered his family and tried to kill himself, allegedly when he was intoxicated with absinthe. The absinthe producers claimed that whilst Lanfray was certainly drunk, absinthe alone could not be blamed for his deeds. They said that Lanfray was a notorious drunkard and that on that fateful day had consumed many other drinks before taking just a couple of glasses of The Green Fairy. No matter, what today would be called a media frenzy, erupted against absinthe and following the outcry, a petition for its ban.

Meanwhile, the wine growers of France had become increasingly disturbed by a dramatic fall in wine production due to nation-wide damage to the roots of the vines by an insect pest, a beetle called phylloxera. There followed a dramatic fall in wine production and a calamitous fall in wine sales which was made much worse by the competition of cheap, mass-produced absinthe.

In an unlikely union, the wine makers allied themselves with the very powerful French temperance movement with the common aim of getting absinthe totally prohibited. It was first banned by the military in the Congo in 1898, then the Netherlands in 1909, Switzerland in 1910, the United States in 1912 and France in 1915 – the French thought that their troops, enfeebled by absinthe-tippling, risked losing World War I to the bellicose, beer-swilling Huns.

Absinthe was never banned in the United Kingdom, but it was never nearly as popular as in France. The British preferred the devils they knew, beer, whisky and gin, to Green Fairies. Remarkably, almost a century after it was totally banned, the Green Fairy has made a comeback in France and on the other side of the English Channel has inspired a cultish devotion among the binge-drinking British youth... who mix absinthe with blackcurrant juice.

BUT WHAT OF THE HIGHLY TOXIC THUJONE? What about the 19th century French doctors who diagnosed absinthisme and who chronicled its symptoms; sudden delirium, epileptic attacks, hallucinations, vertigo, suicidal tendencies? They went as far as claiming it could cause spontaneous human combustion. With such terrible toxic effects how could absinthe ever be restored to the list of respectable drinks?

To the forensic scientists who studied absinthe it became evident that the effects of the low levels of thujone in commercially produced absinthe had been greatly exaggerated. That is not to say that in high doses thujone is not extremely toxic and will produce the alarming symptoms described by the physicians of La Belle Époque.

Analysis of present-day and the original recipes for making absinthe has shown levels of thujone so low that a person would have to drink large quantities of absinthe before exceeding the blood threshold level for thujone toxicity – it just couldn't happen. The quantity of alcohol consumed in the absinthe would render the drinker comatose and he would slip under the table long before achieving a blood concentration sufficient to cause thujone poisoning. Many illegal producers of absinthe in the nineteenth century, however, sold cheap imitations which were contaminated and had higher levels of thujone than commercial absinthe. Those moonshine absinthes could lead to the toxic effects which contemporary physicians diagnosed as absinthisme.

Absinthe was allowed to return to shops and bars in much of Western Europe in 1981 when the European Union overturned the ban. In 1988 the French lifted the ban on absinthe but would allow it to be sold only under the description, *liqueur spiritueuse aux plantes d'absinthe*. In May 2011 the French authorities allowed it to be marketed under its real appellation, absinthe.

AND WHAT ABOUT VINCENT AND HIS ABSINTHISME? Was he poisoned by cheap, illicit absinthe or was he suffering from alcoholism by another name? Was he actually touched by The Green Fairy? His family history suggests that he might have had an extreme sensitivity to thujone related to an inherited metabolic disorder, porphyria – the condition which possibly caused the episodic madness of King George III of England.

It is possible to incriminate one or a mixture of serious ailments as the cause of Vincent's madness. He had epilepsy, but that was probably secondary to his alcoholism. He may have had chronic thujone poisoning from cheap, home-made absinthe. He could have had lead poisoning from his habit of licking his paint brushes to sharpen the tips. His early life was psychologically very disturbed; at one stage he had extreme religious fervour. Some have suggested he had bipolar psychosis (manic depression) others have incriminated syphilis of the nervous system which was common and untreatable in those days – his brother, Theo, was diagnosed as having dementia paralytica (syphilis of the nervous system, General Paresis of the Insane) and died of it at the age of thirty-three, six months after Vincent died.

Shall we ever know the real story? Now that The Green Fairy is back among us, maybe we can experiment with her and after passing a number of green hours in her company she might be persuaded to reveal the true story of Vincent, her troubled devotee.

18. THE MAQUIS OF MONT VENTOUX

RECENTLY THE MAYOR OF OUR LITTLE FRENCH MARKET TOWN at the foot of Mont Ventoux in northern Provence gave my wife an article about the experiences of a foot soldier with the French Resistance in World War II. The soldier, Abraham Felzner, served with the branch of the Resistance, called the Maquis, in the wild and mountainous regions of Vercors, the Drôme and Mont Ventoux.

I translated the article, and because I live so close to Mont Ventoux I felt an immediacy which made me want to know more about the Resistance, more about the Maquis, and that dark epoch in the history of France. As I researched, read, and learned, I was moved to write this essay as a personal tribute to those three hundred and fifty-three young men who lost their lives while fighting for France in the Maquis of Mont Ventoux.

In World War II the French Resistance did not face just one enemy. The German Army and the Gestapo were their principal opponents, they were brutal, but worse were their fellow countrymen, traitors to France who were armed by the Nazi Germans, who volunteered to join a paramilitary militia (the Milice Française) and delighted in doing dirty work for the Nazis. In addition to the Milice there was an abundance of informers who would disclose information about the Resistance for cash; for food, to ingratiate themselves, to settle old scores or to save their own skins.

Members of the Maquis were called Maquisards. For up to four years they endured the harsh winters on the mountains in a state of near-starvation. Although the Maquisards were separated from their families and the comforts of home life for years on end there was worse threatening every member – the prospect of summary execution if captured.

The Resistance represented the noble aspects of the French national character; courage, resourcefulness, daring, and fortitude. Scores of groups of patriots operating independently across the whole country formed the Resistance which eventually became organised under one leader, General Charles de Gaulle, who became the head of the Free French Provisional Government in Exile.

The Maquis of Ventoux was one of the most active divisions of the Resistance. The word maquis is derived from the Italian 'macchia' and translates best as 'brushland.' It was this thick, up to two metres tall, wild land in the lower mountain reaches of Provence, Corsica, and the Vercors that provided sanctuary for the Maquisards. The term maquis probably originated in Corsica when outlaws, feeling that the police were hot on their trail, took to hiding in the brushland; leading to the expression, 'Il a pris le maquis.' – 'He has taken [to] the maquis.'

These days the maquis is best known for the spicy perfume it gives off in spring and summer. Once sniffed, the aroma is never forgotten. Appearing in the spring it is strongest in the heat of summer and comes from the aromatic oils exuded from the leaves of a dozen varieties of plants and small trees.

'THANK GOD FOR THE FRENCH ARMY,' said Winston Churchill in 1933, soon after Adolf Hitler seized power in Germany. Hitler was an inspired leader who at that time was taking his country out of post-World War I feelings of defeatism and fiscal penury and, with remarkable success, restoring German national pride. With evangelistic fervour he convinced Germans that they were the master race and unified nationwide aggression by whipping up hatred of Jews, homosexuals, Freemasons, communists, gypsies, and inferior non-Aryan races.

Churchill was confident. He knew that the French had massive military strength and that the Franco-German border could not be breached. The invincible Maginot Line protected the centre and the south of France and before it reached the Italian border in the Alps the French had erected a chain of well-armed command posts for further protection, in addition to the natural defences offered by the mountainous and hostile terrain. In the north the Ardennes forests provided an impenetrable barrier reaching as far as the Belgian border. In September 1939 at the outbreak of World War II the combined military strengths of the Allies – Britain, France and Poland – numerically exceeded that of Nazi Germany.

Churchill's confidence was to be shattered. The German military was well trained, supremely confident, fanatically motivated, and equipped with modern weapons. Compared with the German military machine the French forces were obsolete. France had lightly armed and slow tanks which were no match for the German Panzer divisions. In pre-emptive strikes the German air force, the Luftwaffe, destroyed half the French air force as it sat on the ground. Surviving French aircraft which took to the skies were easy prey for the brilliant Messerschmitt 109 and Focke-Wulfe 190 fighter aircraft.

The German invasion of France and the Low-Countries unrolled with breathtaking speed, once Hitler's forces entered France on 10 May 1940. On 14 May

Holland surrendered. On 20 May German spearheads reached the English Channel. A week later the Belgian army surrendered. Just before the Germans reached Paris on 9 June the French government fled to Bordeaux. Panzer divisions broke through the impenetrable Ardennes forests and had no need to breach the Maginot Line – they outflanked it.

THE GERMAN BLITZKRIEG RACED ALL OVER THE NORTHERN HALF OF FRANCE. Rapidly advancing ground forces were preceded by Luftwaffe bombers. Hundreds of thousands of desperate, frightened refugees fleeing the cities blocked the roads preventing movement of the French and British military. Their terror was made even worse as they were machine-gunned by fighter aircraft and bombed by Stuka dive bombers. Fitted onto Stukas, and their bombs, were fiendish devices, whistles, which emitted high-pitched screams as the bombers dived and the bombs fell. The screaming, the explosions and the machine gunning further increased the fear of the helpless columns of old, very young and infirm refugees struggling with their precious belongings.

Six weeks and a day after Nazi Germany invaded, France capitulated. The president of the Third Republic, Albert Lebrun, appointed Deputy Prime Minister Marshal Pétain – France's eighty-four year old hero of the First World War – as Prime Minister of the new government.

Hostilities in the First World War had ended by the Germans surrendering on 11 November 1918, and the war was formally concluded by the signing of the Treaty of Versailles on 28 June 1919. The treaty was signed in a railway carriage on the edge of the Forest of Compiègne, by the German military command and witnessed by the French Supreme Commander, Marshal Foch and the Allied General Staff. It included terms which humiliated Germany and imposed crippling reparations. Throughout the First World War the railway carriage had been for

Marshal Foch's personal use. After the war it was employed as a normal carriage on the French railway until system until in 1927 it was returned, as a memorial, to the site of the signing of the armistice.

In World War II, on 22 June 1940, General Charles Huntziger signed the armistice documents on behalf of France; in that same railway carriage and on the exact spot where it had stood on the edge of Compiègne Forest, sixty kilometres north of Paris, twenty-two years before. It gave Hitler great pleasure and satisfaction, but he declined to be a signatory. Hitler sat on the very chair which Marshal Foch had occupied and, after listening to the preamble to the agreement, rose from his seat, gave the Nazi salute, and, in a calculated gesture of contempt to the French delegation left the carriage leaving his chief of staff, General Wilhelm Keitel, to read the terms of the armistice.

Out of interest, it can be told here, that Keitel remained Hitler's right-hand man in military matters throughout the war. Hitler promoted him to field marshal but, because of his constant and irritating toadying to Hitler, the German military elite nicknamed him the Lakeitel, the German for lackey being *lackai*. Keitel was destined to wield his signature at another surrender ceremony almost five years later. On 9 May 1945, ten days after Hitler shot himself and the new Mrs Hitler, née Eva Braun, swallowed a lethal dose of cyanide, Keitel signed the general surrender document ending World War II for Germany. Yet further ignominy awaited him, eighteen months later, when he was found guilty of war crimes at his trial in Nuremberg, he was hanged.

Pétain reorganised the disbanded democratic government of the Third Republic into an authoritarian regime. The new government headquarters was established in the spa town of Vichy in the middle of France. Known as The Vichy Government it was from the start a Nazi puppet. In theory Vichy had authority over the whole of France; in practice Hitler divided the country into two principal zones. France, north of Vichy, became the Occupied Zone ruled by the Wehrmacht (the German army); France south of Vichy together with its overseas territories became the Free Zone, directly administered by the Vichy government. The division lasted until 8 November 1942 when the Allies invaded the North African part of overseas Vichy. Then Hitler, fearing an invasion through the south of France, ordered the Wehrmacht to occupy free Vichy.

A SLIVER OF THE SOUTH EAST OF FRANCE WAS GIVEN TO THE ITALIANS, who had declared war against France and Great Britain exactly a month after the German invasion of France. The leader of the Italian fascist regime, Il Duce, Benito Mussolini, was so dazzled by the successes of the German army and Luftwaffe that he thought that the war would be over in no time. He confided in his Army's Chief of Staff, Marshal Bagdolio, 'I only need a few thousand dead so that I can sit at the peace conference as a man who has fought.'

President Roosevelt of the United States had a different take, 'On this tenth day of June 1940 the hand that held the dagger has struck it into the back of its neighbour.'

Hitler sent one and a half million French soldiers to Germany as forced labourers. To support the three hundred thousand German occupying forces in the north Vichy France was required to pay four hundred million francs a day; fifty times the actual cost.

The Vichy government established its own militia, mostly drawn from the surrendered French army, the Service d'Ordre Legionnaire (SOL) numbering one hundred thousand, which together with sixty thousand gendarmes maintained civil law and order.

In January 1943 another Vichy militia, the Milice Française, was formed; it numbered thirty five thousand. The members were all volunteers and known as Miliciens. Miliciens did not volunteer out of patriotic duty; petty criminals were recruited by promises that their offences would be forgotten; others, whose families had been killed and homes destroyed by Allied bombing, joined out of a sense of grievance and many were attracted by the prospects of regular pay and food to feed their families.

The Milice was a lightly armed paramilitary force which, co-operated with the Gestapo in rounding up Jews, communists, and other undesirables. It supported the German army in its skirmishes with the Maquis. The Milice cultivated informers, participated in summary executions, carried out assassinations, and frequently used torture.

Within months of the surrender of France many of the general population, who had felt it their duty to support Vichy as the legitimate government, became more and more dismayed by its collaboration and subservience to the Nazis. Support for Vichy turned to horror when the harsh treatment meted out by the occupying forces was witnessed. Horror was turned to disgust by the callous activities of their fellow countrymen in the Milice Française. Chronic food shortage was resented with the resentment further fuelled by most of the massive output of French agriculture being sent to Germany at knock-down prices. But it was the conscription of young men for forced labour which triggered the wholesale recruitment into the Resistance and its member group the Maquis.

ABRAHAM FELZNER WAS ONE OF THOSE YOUNG MEN. In 1941 he left the Occupied Zone in Paris to go to the Free Zone in Avignon, fifty kilometres south-west of Mont Ventoux. There he continued his trade as a tailor. One day the Maison de Couture, a tailoring establishment in which he worked, was subjected to a surprise inspection by gendarmes. He was one of half a dozen picked out and ordered to accompany the police to the office of the STO (Service du Travail Obligatoire – the Forced Labour Service). He appealed for a day's grace in order to finish a garment he had begun, this was allowed. Next day he failed to appear, instead he took a bus to Carpentras and then on to Sault, the gathering point for potential maquisards in the Ventoux area.

Sault is a town to the east of Mont Ventoux with the mountains of the Vercors to the north. It is a perched village (village perché), high on the Plateau d'Albion, and nowadays has grown into a typical peaceful Provençal market town. Sault and its surrounding area are known for lavender fields; sheep rearing, pig farming, and nougat.

In World War II Sault was the headquarters of the Ventoux Maquis. After the war the town was awarded the Croix de Guerre in recognition of the valiant role it had played. Sault has easy access to the mountains and forests allowing the maquisards to melt away. The plateau of Albion provided landing strips for parachuted arms containers, radio transmitters and agents flown in from England.

THE VENTOUX MAQUIS WAS COMMANDED BY LIEUTENANT COLONEL BEYNE, a senior tax official based at Sault and a veteran infantry officer of the First World War. He took charge of training and was code named d'Artagnan. His second-in-command, Maxime Fischer from Paris, was a Jewish Parisian lawyer and, like all Jewish lawyers practising in Paris, he had been disbarred. His maquis code name was Anatole. From the many post-war accounts of ex-Ventoux maquisards it is clear that Colonel Beyne and Maxime Fischer commanded the respect and affection of their men.

The Ventoux Maquis numbered about a thousand. They were dispersed around the mountain and into the neighbouring Drôme in units of thirty. Knowing that the maquisards would need new identity cards the prescient Colonel Beyne had the foresight to slip into his pocket official rubber stamps from the town halls he visited in his capacity as a regional tax inspector. Thus he was able to issue the maquisards with false but genuine-looking identity papers, an essential precaution; if they were captured and their true identities were revealed, reprisals would be inflicted on their families.

Abraham Felzner was inducted into the Maquis by Anatole and issued with identity papers bearing the name Albert Fels. Felzner remained in Sault for a few days until he heard that the Gestapo was searching the town; an informer had told the Vichy authorities that maquisard recruits were assembling there. For a few days he and his group hid in an abandoned village in nearby hills but the fear of discovery kept them on the move. Felzner's group of twenty was armed – with five ancient muskets and forty musket-balls stolen from a police station. They existed on food begged from farms and drank ersatz coffee made from toasted barley.

The Maquis worked closely with de Gaulle's Free French Government in London and with the clandestine forces of the British Special Operations Executive (SOE). The SOE was set up to conduct espionage, to train and operate alongside resistance fighters, supply radio transmitters and to arrange parachute drops of arms and agents.

Abraham Felzner became an expert in liaising and conducting operations with the SOE. Operational radio messages were sent from England through the British Broadcasting Company (BBC) and an apparent piece of nonsense like, 'the crow will sing three times in the morning,' could convey vital information. On receipt of notification of a drop Felzner would organise his group and prepare a landing strip on the plateau of Albion. Flares would be lit to guide the incoming aircraft and extinguished as soon as the aircraft, after a few runs, indicated with a flashing red lamp that its load had been discharged.

Felzner preferred it when the British were making the drop because they flew in low. The Americans habitually remained high and that resulted in their parachutes not being concentrated but scattered over several square kilometres; making collection more time-consuming and increasing the likelihood of detection.

On one occasion Felzner led a mission to destroy a transformer in a factory at Sisteron, a town to the east of the Ventoux. Taking plastic explosives and armed with just one Colt revolver Felzner and three others cut their way through a stout metal fence and entered the factory. Under the approving eyes of silent French workers the Maquisards planted the explosives. As they were leaving the workers quietly applauded them. Minutes after they had left they heard the explosion, and then the workers' voices, raised in the Marseillaise.

The Maquis regularly attacked police and military outposts in the Ventoux region; their principal objective was getting arms. They also disrupted communications, cut telephone wires and power cables, destroyed roads and railway tracks which they either blew up or, more economically, caused derailments simply by removing the bolts holding the rails.

Once, travelling along a mountain road, Felzner and his companions came upon a woman walking briskly on her own. Such an unusual occurrence prompted them to arrest her for interrogation. She told them that she was called Cécile Bienkowski and that she was Polish. Suspicions were raised when she could give only vague answers to questions about what she was up to, and so she was held captive. Felzner's group was joined by another group of maquisards which included in its ranks a young man called Max. After several days Cécile went missing and then after another day or two Max disappeared.

A few weeks later, to his surprise, Felzner bumped into Max in the market town of Carpentras. Max explained to Felzner that he had joined another unit of maquisards. Suspicions aroused, Max was tailed. Evidently he was meeting Cécile and passing information to her, which she then relayed to the Milice. Max and Cécile were arrested at their next rendezvous. They were both shot.

Not all groups of ostensible maquisards were genuine. Criminals under the guise of resistance workers terrorised local farmers, stole their livestock and sold it on the thriving black market.

Felzner was ordered by Colonel Beyne to investigate. At one farm, which had been pillaged, not only of sheep but also the jewels of the farmer's wife, he interviewed the farmer but he was too afraid to agree to identify the thieves. He then found a farmer who had been supplying the Maquis with food. This farmer knew the robbers, knew where they were hiding, and was willing to identify them. It was agreed that Felzner would say that he was a butcher and wanted to buy sheep on the black market.

THE MAQUISARDS ARRIVED AT THE CRIMINALS' LAIR in the early morning. There were four, one was shaving with a cut-throat razor and immediately went to attack Felzner, but dropped the razor when a gun was levelled at him. The four were arrested and handed over to the gendarmes in Sault. The youngest of them was a member of an influential family in Carpentras; the gendarmes released him.

On 21 February 1944 Felzner was quartered in a hamlet in the Drôme, Izon-la-Bruisse, with the leaders Colonel Beyne and Captain Maxime. A large contingent, drawn from several groups around Mont Ventoux, was present and morale was exceptionally high. Felzner in his account recorded, 'Joy reigns in the camp. After months and months of deprivation and poverty we are going to eat our fill for once. Each section, after a raid on Buis-les-Baronnies, is going to receive a pig in its rations tomorrow, Mardi Gras.'

Colonel Beyne, Captain Maxime, and other officers with a score of men, walked the few kilometres to the village of Séderon for a conference. They were due to return to Izon-la-Bruisse the next day but shortly before dawn German Wehrmacht forces and the Milice Française attacked. That day thirty-five maquisards were killed, a few in the fighting, but most afterwards... they were summarily executed.

There was one survivor of the group at Izon-la-Bruisse, Laurent Pascal, alias Rolland Perrin. He escaped and survived to give an account of what had happened.

Early in the morning, while he was sleeping in a farm hut and it was still dark, Pascal was woken by a milicien jabbing the muzzle of a sub-machine gun into his belly and saying, 'Get up and don't try to be smart.'

He could do nothing, although his tommy-gun was hanging above him, it was out of reach. As the milicien roughly shoved him through the door of the hut he tripped over something, it was the body of an old friend, Couston.

Pascal was taken to a chapel and thrown inside to join fellow Maquisards already taken. Several hours passed, they discussed their possible fate and questioned how it could have happened that they had suffered such a surprise attack when guards had been posted at key points. Some thought they would be sent to Germany, others feared a worse fate. Pascal took from his pocket a letter he had recently written to his fiancée, Ginette, and in front of all of them tore it into minute fragments so that she could not be incriminated. He suggested to his comrades that they should do the same with any documents they had on their persons.

Suddenly the door flew open and an SS corporal accompanied by two miliciens entered. The corporal demanded to know who was the officer in charge. Pascal stepped forward to explain that none of them officers and that at twenty he was the oldest. He also explained that their officer had slept elsewhere, but that he had no idea where. That appeared to satisfy the German and he and the miliciens left.

Ten minutes later the two miliciens returned and

ordered Pascal outside. They interrogated him, declaring that he knew more than he had admitted. While they were punching and kicking him Pascal spotted two comrades, Cyprien and Noiret, who had disappeared a few days earlier. Now they were smoking cigarettes and chatting with SS officers. During Pascal's beating he lost his shoes and was struck several times with a rifle butt. After an hour he was thrown back with his comrades. When he had recovered he was able to tell them what he had witnessed and thus gave an explanation of how the surprise attack had happened; despite sentries being posted at crucial positions. The maquisard guards had been silently killed before the attack began.

At ten in the morning miliciens forced them out of the chapel at gun point. As they emerged they heard the rattle of small-arms gun fire from above, it was maquisards from a unit called La Forestière, attempting to free them. The miliciens pushed Pascal and his comrades to the front to act as human shields, immediately the firing ceased.

They were taken to a nearby bergerie (sheep farm), the farmer was nowhere to be seen. They learned later that he had been shot by the Germans who then, for amusement, machine-gunned his flock. Two milice brought out a handcart they had found in a barn and ordered Felzner and his companions to throw all their belongings into it. Then they were ordered to march down a hill to the nearby village of Eygalayes.

As they began the descent Pascal saw his comrade and old friend, Marvan, lying on the ground, he had been shot in the foot and could not walk. With permission Pascal hoisted him onto his back and joined what he called in his report, 'the lamentable procession.' The descent was difficult on a snow-covered track, Pascal had no shoes; his blue, naked feet were mocked by the miliciens. He carried the wounded man at the rear of the group of prisoners with the miliciens following closely behind. After ten minutes Pascal was ordered to lower the wounded man to the ground by a milicien who said, 'He will be seen to.'

Pascal knew what would happen. As he lowered him, Marvan begged, 'Do not leave me.'

Pascal had no alternative; he had gone but a couple of metres around a corner when he heard two shots.

An hour after noon a milicien approached the group of maquisards huddling together behind a wall in Eygalayes. He selected four. They were taken behind a farm building; there was a burst of gunfire. Then another milicien appeared for the next four, the same happened. Pascal was in the last quartet, one of whom was a doctor called Toubib. They were pushed around the corner of the building where they saw the bodies of their comrades lying in the blood-spattered snow, two or three moaning as they lay dying.

Pascal looked directly at the milicien standing before him holding a still-smoking sub-machine gun. This fellow Frenchman, a despised collaborator, was to be their executioner. As Pascal glared at him he shifted on his feet, he was uneasy and he looked away. Desperately Pascal gazed around for any avenue of escape, he had to try something. The doctor edged close to him and whispered, 'Now Pascal, get out of here!'

PASCAL DASHED FORWARD, A FRIEND, BLANCHET, WHO LAY mortally injured, had enough strength left to call out and wish him luck. In his report Pascal said, 'Those words of Blanchet gave me wings,' and spurred on, he flew into a field.

He had lost his own shoes during the beating but fortunately he was now wearing a pair of flat shoes he had taken from a dead comrade and which, despite lacking laces, fitted well and clung to his feet. Toubib, the doctor, followed close behind Pascal shielding him with his body. The doctor managed to hold out for about thirty metres, finally staggering and falling as he took bullets aimed at Pascal. Laurent Pascal wrote in his report to Colonel

Beyne, 'I will always have an emotional thought for Toubib, a Jewish doctor of Polish origin, who courageously sacrificed his skin to protect my flight. I am convinced that was his last thought, I most assuredly owe him my life.'

It was a time of great hope in France when the Allies invaded the coast of Normandy on 6 June 1944. The Resistance was well organised and with a strength of a hundred thousand across the country it played an important part in helping the Allies. The Resistance provided intelligence about coastal fortifications and troop movements. It disrupted telecommunications; blew up bridges and railway lines, derailed trains, attacked power stations, fuel depots, arms depots and harassed troop convoys. So successful was the Resistance that the Wehrmacht was frequently unable to move troops in numbers around France. Not only were the railways paralysed by sabotage of the lines, the Resistance destroyed nearly two thousand locomotives.

Ten weeks later the Maquis in the south played the same role as their Resistance comrades in the north. On 15 August the south of France was invaded by Allied Forces which had assembled in Corsica. Corsica had been liberated in September 1943 and served as an allied military base from which air and ground assault forces were launched. Airborne troops in gliders preceded the ground forces which landed by sea on the Côte d'Azur.

Hitler had never regarded the South of France as being of strategic value and the Wehrmacht forces were spread thinly. Some were old and wounded soldiers who had fought on the Eastern Front; others were volunteer battalions from Polish, Czechoslovakian, and even Russian, prisoners of war – not good fighting material. There was just one panzer division south of Vichy.

The Allied commander requested that the Maquis occupy all the villages on the periphery of Mont Ventoux. The Germans defended their positions with no discernible strategy. Motorised units of the Wehrmacht and Miliciens entered the towns of Malaucène and Beaumes de Venise, with what in mind was never clear; but when they left they had killed nine and mortally wounded eight. Similarly they entered Valréas, in the Papal Enclave, where the maquisards had been joined by the town gendarmerie, which had switched sides; together they occupied the town hall and the post office. The maquisards put up stiff opposition in Valréas and achieved signal success, by downing one German fighter aircraft and severely damaging another, by hand-held machine-gun fire.

The maquisards entered the ancient town of Vaison-la-Romaine but were driven out by the occupying German forces. After which the Germans took a hundred civilian hostages and executed twenty five of them.

One thousand two hundred Germans took the town of Nyons in the Drôme. The mayor attempted to talk to the Commandant but he declared that unless resistance stopped immediately he would raze the town. House-to-house searches for arms yielded little; but twenty-six maquisards who had been taken at a road block were marched into the town, lined up against a wall and, together with an equal number of the town's citizens, were shot dead.

Throughout the region the maquisards attacked and harried the German forces which were retreating as fast as they could up the valley of the river Rhône along with the solitary Panzer division. The advance of the Allies in the south was as rapid as that of the Nazi Blitzkrieg through the north of France four years before. So fast was the advance that, within ten days of the landings of the Allies on the coast, the ancient papal city of Avignon was liberated.

On 26 August 1944, when the Allies triumphantly entered and liberated Vaison-la-Romaine, the heroic mission of the Maquis of Mont Ventoux was concluded.

The Supreme Allied Commander, Dwight D.

Eisenhower was fulsome in his praise of the French resistance forces: '…without the French Resistance the liberation of France would have taken much longer and the Allies would have suffered greater losses.'

Scattered around the Ventoux and Drôme are scores of memorials to the memory of Maquisards who died for France… Mort pour la France.

LOCALLY THE FRENCH ARE COMMENDABLY ENTHUSIASTIC IN REMEMBERING the Second World War, the Maquis of Ventoux and the liberation of Provence. Each year my small town, Malaucène, commemorates its liberation. Several American army jeeps, trucks, and military ambulances, all restored to pristine condition, parade around the town. With barbecues in full swing, there is dancing in the main street to the strains of Glen Miller and the townsfolk dress as if they were living in occupied France. Monsieur le Maire becomes a Maquisard wearing a black beret on his head and a holstered pistol at his waist.

The liberation is further commemorated by a memorial and an annual ceremony in a nearby valley where an American P47 Thunderbolt piloted by a Free French officer, Capitaine Joseph Jallier, crashed. The aircraft was flying out of Corsica with a mission to attack Luftwaffe aircraft at a military airfield near Orange.

His approach was from the east, from behind Mont Ventoux. Capitaine Jallier rapidly descended from ten thousand feet and flying low shot up several German aircraft parked on the tarmac. He then turned south, overflew the plain of Carpentras, turned left and once again his approach run began behind Mont Ventoux.

Again he strafed the airfield and turned, but as he was flying away from Orange heading east his Thunderbolt was hit and he progressively lost control as it began its final descent. After staggering along for some forty kilometres in the doomed Thunderbolt, Capitaine Jallier managed to escape from the cockpit, but just as he was jumping the aircraft flipped over and the tailplane struck his head and killed him. The Thunderbolt hit the ground close to Malaucène.

DULCE ET DECORUM EST PRO PATRIA MORI
– it is sweet and glorious to die for one's country
(Horace).

ACKNOWLEDGEMENTS

To Maria, my wife, Stephen, my son, and friends; Maggie Fenton, Dick Gregory, Marc Levillion, Christopher Macrea and Sean Sieck, my thanks for reading some chapters and making suggestions.

BY THE SAME AUTHOR

Bill Larkworthy has written his memoir, *'DOCTOR LARK, the benefits of a medical education.'* Peter Mayle (author A Year in Provence etc.) said it is – 'Interesting and well written … a winner.'

The following introduction will give you a taste of DOCTOR LARK.

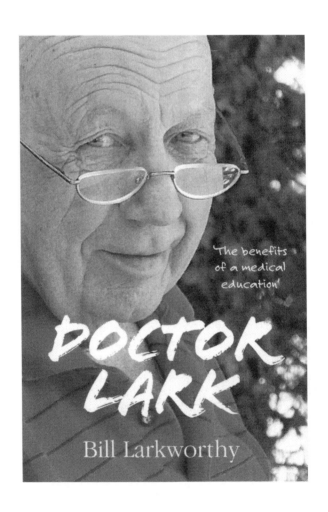

The benefits
of a medical
education

*DOCTOR
LARK*

Bill Larkworthy

INTRODUCTION

ONE BITTERLY COLD WINTER FORTY-FIVE
years ago, I found myself marooned on a nuclear bomber
station on the wind-swept plains of Northern Germany, a
junior doctor in the Royal Air Force.

Christmas celebrations were in full swing and, as the
lowest ranking medical officer, I had been handed the
short straw and was on call for the festive season. This
didn't prevent me from partaking of a large turkey dinner,
or from dozing contentedly afterwards. And sure as a glass
of port follows a good meal, the inevitable happened. I
was summoned by an urgent call: 'Come quickly, sir,
there's been a suicide, there's blood everywhere.'

I dashed and skidded over the icy paths to sick quarters
and forced my way through a knot of airmen who crowded
the entrance, chattering excitedly. A trail of blood led me
to the victim who was in the operating theatre being
cleaned by a couple of orderlies; surprisingly, in view of
the generous quantity of blood splashed about, no source
of bleeding could immediately be found.

Clearly the 'suicide', a mop-headed corporal named
O'Malley, could neither focus nor walk a straight line and
though practically legless, grinned lopsidedly around the
room, not unhappy to be the centre of attention.

We asked one of his mates what had happened. It
seemed O'Malley had been drinking solidly in the
Corporals' Club since Christmas Eve, became maudlin on
Christmas Day, pulled out a penknife on Christmas
afternoon, declared he was going to end it all and set to

work cutting off his thumb. Sure enough, eventually we found a ragged incision on the back of his left thumb. Drunks can bleed profusely but even so, this was barely credible.

'What on earth have you been up to, corporal?' I demanded.

His brow furrowed as he attempted to concentrate and get a fix on my position with wobbly, bleary, bloodshot eyes. He paused, hiccupped, took a deep breath and in an Irish brogue slurred, 'I was depressed, sor, I wanted to kill myself.'

In my supercilious, know-it-all young flight lieutenant doctor's voice I exclaimed, 'But corporal, you don't commit suicide by cutting off your thumb!'

After a moment's reflection he replied: 'Ah well you see, sor, I don't have the benefits of a medical education.'

THAT WAS A LONG TIME AGO, BUT THE STORY has stuck in my mind and led me at times to reflect on the benefits I've had from my medical education. For someone like me from modest origins, the benefits have been many: a fascinating career, a passport to all walks of life, to immense job satisfaction, to friendship and to an adequate income. Not least, because I qualified in 1957, I have witnessed, and participated in, the miraculous developments of the past half-century in medical science and life in general.

'Doctoring', as I thought of it when I was young, has taken me to many far-flung parts of the globe that I might not otherwise have visited. Many of them – Malaysia, Cyprus, Germany, the Persian Gulf – I recall with a fondness bordering on tearful nostalgia while just as many others – Aden, Bangkok, Moose Jaw – have thankfully faded in my memory like a snapshot left too long in the sun.

Much of that travel was courtesy of the Royal Air Force, both by way of overseas postings and the journeys necessitated by the work I was sent there to do. Sometimes it was comfortable, like the mammoth tour of RAF bases between London and Hong Kong by de Havilland Comet. Sometimes it was… less comfortable. Observing terra firma above your head from the seat of a Mirage fighter jet, while flying upside-down is, in my experience, a sure way to nausea.

At least that was a seat and a means of emergency egress, should the need arise. I was singularly unimpressed when I learned that my space in a Canberra bomber – actually a face-to-the-tarmac couchette in the nose of the beast – did not come with the luxury of a parachute. 'Well Bill,' said my ever-helpful flight crew, 'where you are, it will be impossible to get out.' On such occasions, I had to remind myself that I had actually volunteered to go along for the ride.

My medical education also introduced me to a cast of characters and plots richer than those of any costume drama or soap. I met the military equivalent of WAGs, the spouses who had to be repatriated because they couldn't deal with a 'hardship' posting in the sun and warmth of Malta, and at the other end of the scale, Gurkha soldiers who knew real hardship and laughed in its face. They were fighting communists, the insurgents du jour, in the jungle of Malaysia. Even in hospital, sick or wounded, these troopers remained highly disciplined: they would snap to attention under the sheets when I approached if they were too ill to get out of bed.

Across my path have strayed various eccentrics, charlatans, buffoons and braggarts; 'doctors' who weren't what they seemed and unsung heroes who most definitely were; a colleague driven to enlist the services of the Russian Mafia and one of Saddam's 'human shields' who lived to drink another bottle of Dom Perignon. There was even a genuine celebrity, the explorer and writer Sir Wilfred Thesiger, who late in his life was a regular visitor to Dubai. One time I fixed his feet with a scalpel. 'Perfect,' he told me, 'now I'll be able to take that walk in the desert with Charles.' Yes, that Charles.

Medicine carried me into the most glorious, beautiful desert of the Middle East and across the thresholds of palaces of breathtaking opulence in the 'magical' kingdom of Saudi Arabia, to a pinnacle of sorts when I could rightly claim to be 'physician to HM the King'. He was a pleasant and dignified man who was grateful when the treatment I prescribed was a success, quite unlike the megalomaniac, drug-addled hospital director who had me thrown into prison — the lowest point in my career. That's when you find out who your friends are, and I've been fortunate to have collected some good ones, especially in Riyadh.

True, there are some things a medical education didn't teach me, like how to fix a leaking car radiator with the contents of a spice shop (think yellow), an antidote to boredom on the Canadian prairies, or how to distinguish between a taxi and a police car on the sinful streets of Patpong... but that's a story in itself. It did teach me indirectly how to operate a modern fast jet's ejection seat – a skill, not surprisingly, that I have never had call to demonstrate.

DOCTORS COLLECT STORIES AS THEY FOLLOW THEIR CAREERS; it's in the nature of the job. I was amazed, as I compiled this memoir, at what came flooding into my mind, one memory triggering another and stories appearing seemingly out of nowhere. Tales I thought I had forgotten came forward, sometimes with the startling clarity of an ageing brain and sometimes, I admit, with embellishments of half-remembered events – well, anyway, this is my life, this is how it looked to me – and it's how I made the most of my medical education...

DOCTOR LARK – the benefits of a medical education is available on Amazon as a paperback and in Amazon Kindle Books.

Printed in Great Britain
by Amazon

48222940R00129